NURSING PRAXIS

NURSING PRAXIS

Knowledge and Action

SALLY E. THORNE
VIRGINIA E. HAYES
editors

SAGE Publications
International Educational and Professional Publisher
Thousand Oaks London New Delhi

For information address:

SAGE Publications, Inc.
2455 Teller Road
Thousand Oaks, California 91320
E-mail: order@sagepub.com

SAGE Publications Ltd.
6 Bonhill Street
London EC2A 4PU
United Kingdom

SAGE Publications India Pvt. Ltd.
M-32 Market
Greater Kailash I
New Delhi 110048 India

Printed in the United States of America

Library of Congress Cataloging-in-Publication Data

Main entry under title:

Nursing praxis: Knowledge and action / editors, Sally E. Thorne &
Virginia E. Hayes.
p. cm.
Includes bibliographical references and index.
ISBN 0-7619-0010-1 (cloth). — ISBN 0-7619-0011-X (pbk.)
1. Nursing—Practice. 2. Nursing—Philosophy. 3. Nursing-
-Research. I. Thorne, Sally E. (Sally Elizabeth), 1951- .
II. Hayes, Virginia E. (Virginia Ellen)
RT86.7.N92 1997
610.73—dc20 96-25360

97 98 99 00 01 02 10 9 8 7 6 5 4 3 2 1

Acquiring Editor: Dan Ruth
Editorial Assistant: Jessica Crawford
Production Editor: Sanford Robinson
Production Assistant: Karen Wiley
Typesetter/Designer: Danielle Dillahunt
Indexer: Cristina Haley
Cover Designer: Lesa Valdez

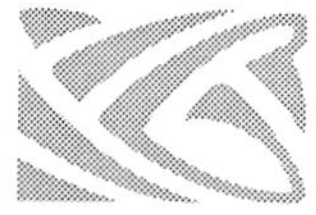

Contents

PART II. APPLIED THEORETICAL KNOWLEDGE

PART III. EMANCIPATORY INQUIRY

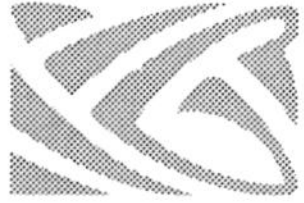

Acknowledgments

The genesis of this book can be traced to two significant events that took place at the University of British Columbia School of Nursing. The first was the long-overdue inauguration of one of the first nursing doctoral programs in Canada (in 1991), which attracted students with voracious appetites for socially relevant knowledge, eager to challenge the limits of their discipline. The second was the highly successful International Nursing Research Conference, held in Vancouver in May 1994, which brought together thinkers and scholars from all corners of the globe, many of whom are working within nontraditional domains linking philosophy, practice knowledge, and science. Inspired by the enthusiasm of both students and experts for such intellectual challenges, and recognizing that the praxis literature is still in its infancy in our discipline, we launched the plan for this collection.

The chapters included in this volume are all invited submissions representing diverse perspectives within practical, theoretical, and academic nursing. The authors agreed to develop their thinking in correspondence with us over the course of a year, and an initial version of each chapter was subject to a critical review by recognized experts in the field prior to final revision.

We are deeply indebted to the authors for their participation in the project and for their commitment to the idea of such a collection. With them, we acknowledge the generous contributions of the expert reviewers, many of whose thoughtful commentaries were themselves of stellar quality and made us wish we had reserved additional space for them in the final publication. Our thanks go to the following reviewers:

Marianne Arndt, Humboldt Universität, Berlin
Ann Bishop, Lynchburg College, Virginia
Claire Budgen, Okanagan University College, Kelowna, British Columbia
Joan Ford, University of Alberta
Barbara Keddy, Dalhousie University
Elizabeth Lindsey, University of Victoria
Juliene Lipson, University of California, San Francisco
Marilyn Mardiros, University of Ottawa
Marjorie McIntyre, University of Calgary
Ellen Olshansky, University of Washington
Barbara Paterson, University of British Columbia
Anneli Sarvimäki, University of Helsinki, Finland
John Scudder, Jr., Lynchburg College, Virginia
Patricia Stevens, University of Wisconsin—Milwaukee
Jan Storch, University of Calgary
Donna Wells, University of Toronto
Judith Wuest, University of New Brunswick

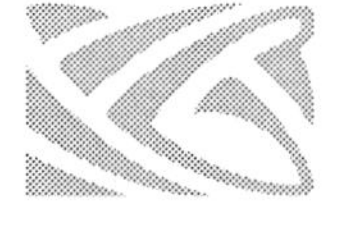

Introduction

Praxis in the Context of Nursing's Developing Inquiry

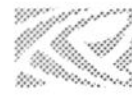

SALLY E. THORNE

NURSING SCHOLARSHIP IN MOTION

Nursing scholarship is in revolution. Despite its self-conscious entry into scientific and academic communities only a few decades ago, nursing has emerged with a distinct voice in the world of ideas. It has developed certain areas of singular credibility, and it has spearheaded important challenges to the accepted scientific "truths" upon which social and health policy has been grounded (Thompson, 1985). The progress of scholarship within nursing can be attributed to the agility with which nursing's leaders have been able to tackle the increasing complexities and ambiguities inherent in human and health sciences, sciences that attempt to unravel the mysteries of human experience in the face of adversity, transformation, and unique meaning (Watson, 1995).

Advances in nursing science reveal an increasingly sophisticated understanding that the cells and organs from which people are constructed represent a very limited perspective on human experience, and that human health and illness must be appreciated in the context of the intellectual and spiritual qualities that make people individuals, the interactions that make them social beings, and the strategies that permit them to live their lives in complex organizational structures (Coppa, 1993). The imperatives of a practice discipline have forced nursing scholars to recognize that ideas are value-laden and have implications that must be considered and managed responsibly (Liaschenko, 1993; Yeo, 1989). Although grand theories might be crafted in relation to aggregates and on the basis of population norms, they must always be applied at the level of individual instances of human experience. Because application within a practice discipline invariably requires judgment about the implications inherent in infinite variation, nurses have had little tolerance for the kind of violent theoretical debate that has characterized some of the social sciences throughout this century. It can be argued that this practice mandate may have been among the factors forcing nursing to escape the bonds of traditional positivism, to forge links between theory and practice, and to tolerate challenges to traditional scientific conventions and methods long before other disciplines were willing to abide rebellions within their science (Reed, 1995).

Ironically, the historically gendered nature of nursing may also have contributed to early successes in "new paradigm" scholarship. As a predominantly female profession, nursing has experienced as much difficulty gaining credibility in the traditional halls of scientific discourse as in the boardrooms of health service delivery. Arguably, then, nursing may have had little to lose in breaking ranks and challenging the status quo in science, practice, and epistemology. Already frustrated by gender and scientific oppression, nursing may have had some advantage over other practice sciences in intuitively appreciating the possibilities inherent in new ways of thinking about knowledge and society (Doering, 1992). As critical social theory, poststructuralism, and feminism were worked out in other disciplines, nurses began to grasp the potential they might offer for challenging the existing order and authenticating the worth of new knowledge sources and inquiry methods (Allen, 1991; Anderson, 1991; Butterfield, 1990; Campbell & Bunting, 1991).

For the past decade or more, nursing has demonstrated leadership within the health disciplines (and some of the social sciences) in developing and refining qualitative approaches to rigorous, scientific research. Far more quickly than has been the case in many other disciplines, mainstream nursing accepted the value of inquiry into subjective human experience in a naturalistic context. Further, it recognized the value of such scholarship beyond mere description and supported the development of considerable substantive theory on the basis of such research. Although some of the early discourse was characterized by a "qualitative versus quantitative" debate, the leaders in nursing science readily accepted the inherent value of embracing multiple approaches to scholarship (Dzurec, 1989). They also began to articulate the urgency of refining a coherent sense of the discipline that makes room for a range of activities and forces scientists to locate their work within philosophical and scientific contexts, rather than assuming such contexts will be understood. As a result of these trends, nurses have informed themselves quite widely in the scholarly traditions of the disciplines from which those original qualitative methods evolved and have developed sufficient confidence to begin to work out modifications and applications of many methodological conventions.

THE NOTION OF PRAXIS

Recent trends further suggest that nurses are increasingly interested not only in theory, practice, and research in isolation, but in various permutations and combinations of these (Kim, 1993; Reed, 1995). Further, they have been attracted by the notion (derived from the concept of praxis) that each of these can inform the others to produce powerful new forms of knowledge (Moccia, 1986). The advent of the concept of "praxis" within nursing signifies that nursing scholarship has taken a turn beyond the preparation of scientists, theoreticians, and practitioners, toward preparation of those who are capable of handling the implications of their ideas within each of these realms (Owen-Mills, 1995). Critical thinking within the discipline takes us beyond concern for which ideas are defensible, in the sense of which ideas can be soundly argued, toward a more complex question: What are the implications of holding certain ideas? Although nursing draws inspiration from fields of scholarship with ancient roots that determine, at least in part, which problems are resolvable and which are not, its practical art and science mandates shift the focus toward an obligation to reconsider those theoretical and philosophical positions in an emancipatory light (Silva, Sorrell, & Sorrell, 1995).

One model of praxis that has gained considerable popularity within nursing is the notion of reflection upon practice toward the refinement of theory and therefore the enhancement of practice. Reflection is understood as a means by which the individual nurse uses the unique conditions of particular cases to challenge and refine the theoretical notions that provide direction for decision making in practice (Mitchell, 1995). This idea can be traced to the seminal work of Benner (1984), who uncovered this form of analysis in the reasoning of expert nursing practitioners. Applications of the idea have mushroomed in popularity, to the point where entire curricula for preparing neophyte nurses are based upon it (Diekelmann, 1995; Perry & Moss, 1989). Although superficial treatments hold that all reflection will inherently produce knowledge for practice, a more critical analysis reveals that Benner's original work (conducted with individuals who had already achieved expertise in practice) betrays a considerably more conservative orientation to knowledge production in context (Cash, 1995). In addition, some authors point out that reflective processes can also entrench prejudices more deeply, reinforce systematic errors in thinking, or otherwise confound the progress of enlightened thinking (Burnard, 1995; Richardson, 1995). That practice scholars recall using the technique toward their development of expertise does not assure us that reflection represents the entire basis for expert knowledge. As many have recognized, expert practice knowledge can also be attributed to a systematic base of thinking (theory), a substantive formal knowledge (including science), and certain critical thinking skills as foundations upon which reflective thinking produces expert practice (Benner, Tanner, & Chesla, 1996; Paul & Heaslip, 1995). It seems quite likely that the value of appreciating a dialectic between thought and action, between knowledge and values, between science and opinion, becomes apparent only when each of the components has achieved a certain level of sophistication (Clarke, James, & Kelly, 1996; Greenwood, 1993; Roy, 1995).

Another domain in which praxis theory has emerged in our discourse is in the trend toward emancipatory research methodologies. Such methods challenge traditional qualitative and quantitative approaches as agents of the status quo and embed normative rather than simply descriptive objectives into our research efforts. Of course, such inquiry demands an explicit acknowledgment of a socially valued and desired outcome, a prior agreement on the nature of a constructive social change. As we know, mechanisms for social consensus or other forms of collective decision toward valued objectives are elusive at best and utterly unattainable at worst, and so scholars in the emancipatory project draw upon a number of frameworks and orientations as guides for their action and knowledge development. Perspectives such as critical theory, feminism, and postmodernism figure prominently in the works of those explicitly associating their theoretical efforts with emancipatory action. Scholars applying these traditions must continuously examine and reflect upon the manner in which the orientation shapes the knowledge they develop in an understanding that such knowledge is a highly social construction, and not knowledge in the traditional factual sense. The efforts of scholars working at the edges of emancipatory inquiry are reflective of nursing action writ large in that they capitalize upon the tension arising from a dialectic among theory, science, and action. At the same time they whittle away at our epistemological foundations, they provide us with new visions of what knowledge can look like, as well as what social and political impacts it might have (Allen, 1992; Holmes, 1993; Kendall, 1992; Stevens, 1989).

THE PRAXIS PROJECT

Nursing scholarship is therefore poised to extend its reach beyond those problems that have been well studied and developed, and into the realm of the unknown. The recent literature resounds with the call to break down the barriers between research and practice, between palliation and prevention, between objectivity and critical thought, between cause and effect, between "researchable problems" and those immense predicaments that threaten the health of the planet and its occupants. This book is an attempt to extend the preliminary discussion that already exists in the literature to illustrate the strength and complexity inherent in the praxis project within nursing. It is intended to counter the current trend toward oversimplification and to make explicit the larger implications of the issues underlying the tension between thought and action. The authors contributing to this book represent nurse philosophers, scientists, and practitioners from diverse backgrounds who share a common proclivity toward inquiry beyond the narrow confines of tradition. Because many take critical positions with regard to the implications of ideas, the reader will note a trend toward dealing not only with processes themselves, but also with outcomes, toward striving to tackle the very difficult and problematic philosophical challenge of "Toward what purpose?"

The contributors to this volume take a range of positions on questions relating to the larger social context within which nursing and scholarship take place. Beyond explicit feminist or critical social positions, the chapters within this book illustrate more generic notions, such as empowerment, the larger social good, and universal values. Although each issue exemplifies a complex philosophical disputation in and of itself, these authors share a conviction that the implications of our uniquely applied discipline add meaningful dimensions to the general discourse of our colleagues from other disciplines. Further, they would contend that the process of such inquiry is in and of itself inherently meaningful within nursing, regardless of whether universal understandings about the larger social good emerge.

Each chapter in this collection tackles practical, philosophical, and professional questions arising from a unique dimension of the dialectic among research, theory, and practice within nursing. In Part I, which is devoted to knowledge in the clinical encounter, the contributors examine a range of issues that emerge when reflectively derived practice knowledge is brought into theoretical perspective.

In Chapter 1, Johnson and Ratner explore the nature of the knowledge that is used in nursing practice, providing a historical and developmental perspective on what counts as knowledge and how we can understand the operations of nursing knowledge over time. In so doing, these authors illuminate and revisit many of the trends that have been apparent and the perspectives they have represented, in essence helping us to deconstruct the claims of our theoretical history. Their thoughtful location of the positions of key thinkers within the theoretical arm of the discipline helps orient us to the traditions embedded in current arguments about various forms and manifestations of knowledge for nursing. They provide us with a heuristic means for classifying knowledge sources and clarifying our discourse about the nature of nursing knowledge.

Liaschenko, in Chapter 2, dives beneath the surface of the call to "know the patient" and orients us to what this might mean for considering the individual as case, patient, or person. Her careful analyses of the contexts in which knowing the patient has been argued reveal the complexities inherent in the enterprise and lead us to critical examination of ways in which knowing the patient might not serve the interests of individuals, nursing, or, indeed, society. Liaschenko's contribution is an orientation to the philosophical positions implied by claims about knowing the patient and a critical social interpretation of what adherence to that value might mean.

Griffin's discussion in Chapter 3 of structural, communicative, cultural, and social knowledge arising from the daily imperatives of a nurse practitioner's work epitomizes the voice of reflective practice in action. Griffin takes the position that practice can and must inform both theory and research if nursing is to contribute to the health of those it serves. In particular, she explicitly illustrates ways in which culture and poverty challenge practitioners to shape their practice action and inform policy.

In her examination of the domain of family nursing in Chapter 4, Hayes finds little evidence of a praxis orientation to knowledge development. She argues for thoughtful consideration of the origins of theoretical applications used by family nurse practitioners and develops a range of strategies by which the knowledge embedded in family nursing practice can be uncovered, considered, and developed. Hayes contends that the substantive field of family nursing is unlikely to advance significantly until a dialectic between theoretical and practical knowledge can be established in the discourse on family nursing.

In Chapter 5's exploration of the intricate interactions between humans and machines, Sandelowski considers technology as an inadequately understood form of knowing within nursing practice, and one that has been entirely invisible in the theoretical debates on sources of nursing knowledge. In recognizing that technology extends the sensory and interpretive capacities of the human user in predictable ways, Sandelowski orients us to moral questions imposed upon us by our technological capacities.

The contributions in Part II are concerned with applied theoretical knowledge within nursing. In Chapter 6, Trainor explicates her point of view that autonomous knowledge development in nursing derives from authority within the discipline to be professional and that enlightenment emerges from philosophic agreements between individual professionals and the aggregate of the discipline. She sees nursing practice and thought as inextricably linked within our social and historical context, and challenges us toward an enlightenment that assures the continuation of our knowledge development through the questioning of authority.

In Chapter 7, Halldórsdóttir reflects upon the act of nursing embodied in the nurse-patient relationship and characterized as "caring." From Halldórsdóttir's perspective, the urgency within theoretical nursing to reconstruct nursing as a phenomenon of caring has sometimes precluded a serious examination of the complexities inherent in professional caring acts, resulting in inadequate definitions to guide and evaluate professional practice. Her inquiries into the perspectives of consumers of professional caring challenge nursing to make its competencies explicit within a moral/ethical relational context.

Locating her work in another dichotomously articulated nursing challenge, Jones examines in Chapter 8 the relationship between theory and practice in shaping clinical knowledge. She contends that an artificially constructed theory-practice gap renders the praxis of nursing invisible. On the basis of her research and analysis, Jones proposes ways in which nurses might be encouraged to "think nursing" in their practice and ways in which the structure and organization of nursing can create conditions that foster integration of thought and action.

In Chapter 9, Miller orients us to the history and traditions of the various postmodern and feminist perspectives that have been applied to nursing theorizing and to the consideration of nursing problems. On the basis of her critical analysis of the implications of these perspectives, Miller offers explicit examples of how postmodern feminist thinking can uncover epistemological contradictions within nursing science, practice, and theory and thereby enlighten the processes of our ongoing inquiry.

Henderson illustrates an application of one form of enlightenment to nursing practice problems in Chapter 10. Her examination of consciousness-raising as a feminist nursing action traces its historical development within the critical social and feminist movements. Henderson argues that nursing has paid insufficient attention to enlightenment, empowerment, and emancipation, and she explores some of the difficulties inherent in the application of these perspectives by practitioners and researchers. She concludes with the contention that consciousness-raising is not only justifiable but also essential within nursing action, and she suggests ways to enact it at the individual and collective level.

In her consideration in Chapter 11 of theoretical applications in the educational domain, Varcoe critically examines the curriculum-as-praxis discourse that has dominated recent nursing education scholarship. She takes the position that reflection and action in the curriculum revolution have focused on the educational context rather than the object of nursing education. Without an emancipatory direction and a client orientation, Varcoe argues, a caring curriculum can perpetuate the inherent domination of both clients and nurses within the health care system.

The discussion shifts in Part III toward an explicit treatment of emancipatory inquiry within knowledge development. In Chapter 12, Maxwell surveys the philosophical foundations upon which nursing's emancipatory research and formal inquiry methods have been based. Locating emancipatory nursing research within an ancient tradition concerned with knowledge for social change, she articulates the roles of such thinkers as Rousseau, Marx, Freire, and

Habermas in guiding our orientation toward inequities in the health context and in directing the mandate of nurse scholars toward socially transformative knowledge.

Starzomski and Rodney, in Chapter 13, tackle the challenging question of how we determine the normative object of inquiry within a discipline such as nursing. Examining the relationship between nursing theory and nursing ethics, these authors consider the implications of various theoretical perspectives for such critical imperatives as health policy and social activism. They conclude that nursing's theoretical work has thus far provided insufficient direction for social, environmental, and political thinking within the discipline, and that attention to the common good, moving our theorizing beyond the individual to the level of the aggregate, must be embedded in all of our analyses.

In Chapter 14, Angerami and Correia offer their perspective on what reflection and action can mean in the broadest context of global health promotion. Their analysis of nursing's role in health issues from the foundation of social responsibility and justice demonstrates how the imperatives most acutely felt by those in the developing world ought to be of concern throughout the discipline. According to the worldview of these authors, reflection and action must occur at levels far beyond the interaction between individual health care providers and recipients; we must consider health issues in the context of populations, societies, and political structures. Angerami and Correia believe that much of our difficulty in apprehending the deeper moral responsibility associated with a global perspective on health issues arises from our capacity to detach our gaze from "the other" and to find comfort within our restricted domains of influence. Thus their chapter represents a moral clarion call for all nurses interested in reflection and action, and for all who claim an emancipatory objective, to consider their ideas within the broadest context of a globally integrated system.

In Chapter 15, Rasmussen addresses the application of action research methodology as both a technique whereby nurses and patients can collaborate to effect change and as a method through which the study of nursing can be advanced. Rasmussen familiarizes us with the history and tradition underlying those research methods we now recognize as having an action orientation and links the moral imperative of those methods with a socially mandated discipline such as nursing. Her discussion makes explicit the kinds of nursing problems that action research can help us to solve.

In the final chapter, McCormick and Roussy assert that postmodernist thought without an emancipatory orientation is problematic for the discipline of nursing. Because of this, they encourage nurse scholars to consider the advantages feminist poststructuralism offers for an appreciation of credible future directions in nursing research, theory, and practice. Surveying current claims about what exists and what the theoretical options might be, these authors address the lived realities and social inequities for which such critical perspectives can offer normative possibilities and permit nursing action toward social change.

Although issues of research methods, theory development, and practice mandate have traditionally been considered in isolation from each other, and many nurse scholars are only marginally comfortable in more than one of these arenas, the thinkers contributing to this book provide evidence that the parallel trends within our disciplinary discourse reflect a larger pattern that demands integrated and comprehensive inquiry. Although knowledge and information proliferation have effectively exceeded the capacity of individuals to be fully expert in domains beyond subspecialties within a discipline, there is a pressing urgency for nurse scholars to dissolve disciplinary boundaries, to explore ideas and methods outside their own safe territories, and to take risks in linking ideas that are complex, highly abstract, and solidly embedded within various traditions.

The chapters within this book illustrate some of the many ways in which nurse scholars are critically reflecting on new approaches, proposing new associations, and pressing nursing science and philosophy ever forward. Changing the angle of vision by considering practice from the perspective of research, theory from the perspective of science, and knowledge from the perspective of action is the embodiment of praxis within nursing. A praxis orientation toward the dialectic between knowledge and action forces us to abandon simple solutions and straightforward answers as we reframe our discipline's fundamental philosophical and social imperatives.

REFERENCES

Allen, D. G. (1991). Critical social theory and nursing education. In N. Greenleaf (Ed.), *Curriculum revolution: Refining the student-teacher relationship* (pp. 546-565). New York: National League for Nursing.

Allen, D. G. (1992). Feminism, relativism, and the philosophy of science: An overview. In J. L. Thompson, D. G. Allen, & L. Rodrigues-Fisher (Eds.), *Critique, resistance, and action: Working papers in the politics of nursing* (pp. 1-19). New York: National League for Nursing.

Anderson, J. M. (1991). Current directions in nursing research: Toward a poststructuralist and feminist epistemology. *Canadian Journal of Nursing Research, 23*(3), 1-3.

Benner, P. (1984). *From novice to expert: Excellence and power in clinical nursing practice.* Menlo Park, CA: Addison-Wesley.

Benner, P., Tanner, C. A., & Chesla, C. A. (1996). *Expertise in nursing practice: Caring, clinical judgement, and ethics.* New York: Springer.

Burnard, P. (1995). Nurse educators' perceptions of reflection and reflective practice: A report of a descriptive study. *Journal of Advanced Nursing, 21,* 1167-1174.

Butterfield, P. G. (1990). Thinking upstream: Nurturing a conceptual understanding of the society context of health behavior. *Advances in Nursing Science, 12*(2), 1-8.

Campbell, J. C., & Bunting, S. (1991). Voices and paradigms: Perspectives on critical and feminist theory in nursing. *Advances in Nursing Science, 13*(3), 1-15.

Cash, K. (1995). Benner and expertise in nursing: A critique. *International Journal of Nursing Studies, 32,* 527-534.

Clarke, B., James, C., & Kelly, J. (1996). Reflective practice: Reviewing the issues and refocussing the debate. *International Journal of Nursing Studies, 33,* 171-180.

Coppa, D. F. (1993). Chaos theory suggests a new paradigm for nursing science. *Journal of Advanced Nursing, 18,* 985-991.

Diekelmann, N. (1995). Reawakening thinking: Is traditional pedagogy nearing completion? *Journal of Nursing Education, 34,* 195-196.

Doering, L. (1992). Power and knowledge in nursing: A feminist poststructuralist view. *Advances in Nursing Science, 14*(4), 24-33.

Dzurec, L. C. (1989). The necessity for and evolution of multiple paradigms for nursing research: A poststructuralist perspective. *Advances in Nursing Science, 11*(4), 69-77.

Greenwood, J. (1993). Reflective practice: A critique of the work of Argyris and Schön. *Journal of Advanced Nursing, 18,* 1183-1187.

Holmes, C. A. (1993). Praxis: A case study in the depoliticization of methods in nursing research. *Scholarly Inquiry for Nursing Practice, 7,* 3-12.

Kendall, J. (1992). Fighting back: Promoting emancipatory nursing actions. *Advances in Nursing Science, 15*(2), 1-15.

Kim, H. S. (1993). Identifying alternative linkages among philosophy, theory and method in nursing science. *Journal of Advanced Nursing, 18,* 793-800.

Liaschenko, J. (1993). Feminist ethics and cultural ethos: Revisiting a nursing debate. *Advances in Nursing Science, 15*(4), 71-81.

Mitchell, G. J. (1995). Reflection: The key to breaking with tradition. *Nursing Science Quarterly, 8*(2), 57.

Moccia, P. (1986). The dialectic as method. In P. L. Chinn (Ed.), *Nursing research methodology: Issues and implications* (pp. 147-156). Rockville, MD: Aspen.

Owen-Mills, V. (1995). A synthesis of caring praxis and critical social theory in an emancipatory curriculum. *Journal of Advanced Nursing, 21,* 1191-1195.

Paul, R. W., & Heaslip, P. (1995). Critical thinking and intuitive practice in nursing. *Journal of Advanced Nursing, 22,* 40-47.

Perry, J., & Moss, C. (1989). Generating alternatives in nursing: Turning curriculum into a living process. *Australian Journal of Advanced Nursing, 6*(2), 35-40.

Reed, P. G. (1995). A treatise on nursing knowledge development for the 21st century: Beyond postmodernism. *Advances in Nursing Science, 17*(3), 70-84.

Richardson, R. (1995). Humpty Dumpty: Reflection and reflective nursing practice. *Journal of Advanced Nursing, 21,* 1044-1050.

Roy, C. L. (1995). Developing nursing knowledge: Practice issues raised from four philosophical perspectives. *Nursing Science Quarterly, 8*(2), 79-85.

Silva, M. C., Sorrell, J. M., & Sorrell, C. D. (1995). From Carper's patterns of knowing to ways of being: An ontological philosophical shift in nursing. *Advances in Nursing Science, 18*(1), 1-13.

Stevens, P. E. (1989). A critical social reconceptualization of environment in nursing: Implications for methodology. *Advances in Nursing Science, 11*(4), 56-68.

Thompson, J. L. (1985). Practical discourse in nursing: Going beyond empiricism and historicism. *Advances in Nursing Science, 7*(4), 59-71.

Watson, J. (1995). Postmodernism and knowledge development in nursing. *Nursing Science Quarterly, 8*(2), 60-64.

Yeo, M. (1989). Integration of nursing theory and nursing ethics. *Advances in Nursing Science, 11*(3), 33-42.

PART I

Knowledge in the Clinical Encounter

1

The Nature of the Knowledge Used in Nursing Practice

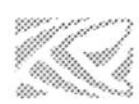

JOY L. JOHNSON
PAMELA A. RATNER

In its broadest sense, the term *praxis* refers to practical human conduct. This conduct can include artistic, ethical, and political activity. One central issue relevant to the realm of praxis concerns the kind of knowledge used in practical human conduct. In that nursing is a form of praxis, questions regarding the nature of the knowledge required for this praxis are central to the nursing discipline. These epistemological questions center on matters such as how the knowledge used in nursing practice is developed and how it is applied. Accordingly, these questions have profound implications for the development of the nursing discipline and the education of nursing professionals. In this chapter, we explore the nature of the knowledge used in nursing practice and highlight several salient epistemological questions that have not been fully explored in the nursing literature.[1] We begin by considering the development of ideas concerning the nature of the knowledge used in nursing practice.

To provide the reader with a point of orientation and a fair opportunity to judge the positions presented, and to avoid any unnecessary ambiguity, we offer the following definitions. For purposes of this chapter, we define *knowledge* very broadly as things perceived or held in consciousness, justified in some way, and therefore regarded as "true" (Angeles, 1981).[2] We recognize that the knowledge used in nursing practice may be subjective or objective. By *subjective knowledge,* we mean knowledge of particulars possessed only by individuals, knowledge that cannot be shared. By *objective knowledge,* we mean knowledge that is generalizable and that can be shared with others. For example, my immediate knowledge of this cold draft in my office that is blowing on my legs is mine alone, and you cannot know what I feel. I can describe the draft to you, but when I do so, I describe it in general or objective terms; this objective knowledge can be shared and commonly understood. Further, the knowledge used to guide nursing practice may be speculative, practical, or both. By *speculative knowledge,* we mean knowledge of what is the case (know-that knowledge); by *practical knowledge,* we mean knowledge of what can be or ought to be done or made (know-how knowledge).[3]

HISTORICAL BACKGROUND

The consideration of the knowledge required for nursing practice has attracted the attention of nursing scholars since the beginning of the modern era of nursing. As the profession of nursing has evolved, so too has the thinking about what constitutes the knowledge used in the conduct of nursing. To place the discussion regarding the nature of the knowledge used in nursing practice within an appropriate context, we briefly trace in this section some conceptual roots of this knowledge, beginning with the work of Florence Nightingale. Our review is not comprehensive, and many important nursing theorists are excluded. We merely aim to highlight some notable distinctions in several nursing theorists' conceptualizations.

Nightingale was firmly committed to the notion that nursing is not an innate ability, but a calling that requires both knowledge and skill. She recognized that, because of their social position and the inadequacies of the contemporary health care system, many women of her time were required to provide nursing care. However, she did not espouse the idea that nursing is synonymous with womanhood: "It has been said and written scores of times, that every woman makes a good nurse. I believe, on the contrary, that the very elements of nursing are all but unknown" (Nightingale, 1860/1969, p. 8). She not only believed that nursing knowledge is learned, but we find in her work the view that the knowledge necessary for nursing practice is derived from three sources. Her curriculum for nursing education was grounded in the basic sciences of biology, anatomy, and hygiene. However, for Nightingale (c. 1899), experience was the sine qua non of knowledge development: "In all things, however, be not satisfied with thinking, do: by doing, and accurately observing at once, experience is gained. By thinking only, ideal theories are gained, brought to the test of no experience, and generally far astray" (quoted in Palmer, 1983, p. 231). Thus, according to Nightingale, two realms of knowledge necessary for practice consist of the basic sciences and the personal insights and skills gained through experience. The third domain of knowledge necessary for practice is said to be the domain of rules. Indeed, much of Nightingale's work focused on detailing procedures for the care of patients. These rules or procedures are putatively based on scientific principles and are inviolable and incontrovertible (Nightingale, c. 1899). In Nightingale's view, three separate realms of knowledge are necessary for nursing practice: the speculative, which is purely objective in that it is derived from the basic sciences, and two practical realms, one consisting of rules and the other consisting of the insights or skills gained through experience.

Isabel Maitland Stewart viewed the knowledge necessary for nursing practice in a light different from that of Nightingale. Rather than seeing experience as foundational to nursing practice, Stewart emphasized that nursing rests on scientific knowledge, which provides the basis for sound nursing practice. She wrote, "The next requirement is *an adequate body of knowledge.* I place this before skill because there can be no safe and intelligent practice without a knowledge of guiding principles. The art or doing side of any work must have sound thinking to back it up, otherwise it becomes merely automatic, rule-of-thumb routine" (Stewart, Clayton, & Jamme, 1916, p. 324). Similarly, Annie

Goodrich (1912) argued that nursing is a profession that possesses special speculative knowledge. Like Nightingale, Stewart and Goodrich believed that knowledge gained through experience alone is not sufficient for nursing practice. However, they held that a balance is necessary between what they saw as an inordinate emphasis placed on experience in the nurses' training schools based on Nightingale's model and the accentuation of formal classroom instruction found in college education (Stewart, 1922). Objective knowledge was believed to inform nursing practice and to help nurses solve particular problems, and was to be used in conjunction with technical skill gained through practice and experience. Goodrich and Stewart saw the roots of the knowledge necessary for nursing practice as arising from two sources: scientifically derived nursing theory and experientially derived skill and technique.

Nurses' quest for professional legitimacy intensified through the mid-1900s, and nursing academicians, in an attempt to portray nursing as a legitimate discipline rightly placed within institutions of higher learning, began to minimize the importance of the technical and experiential aspects of nursing. By the mid-1960s, many nursing theorists supported the view that learned professions and technical work are incompatible. Martha Rogers (1961), for example, asserted that professional nursing is characterized by "essentially intellectual operations" (p. 10) rather than technical operations. Similarly, Mildred Montag (1951) distinguished the "technical nurse," so named because a technician can be defined as one skilled in a practical art, from the professional nurse. So began an intensive search for the theoretical underpinnings of nursing practice.

The search was arguably most ardent in the late 1960s and 1970s, when authors such as Dickoff, James, and Beckstrand sought to articulate the knowledge necessary for nursing practice—what became known as practice theory. Dickoff and James (1968) argued that a practice discipline must develop theory that guides and shapes reality so that the profession's purpose is attained; they referred to this particular kind of theory as "situation-producing." They argued that descriptive or speculative knowledge is not sufficient for nursing practice. The ingredients of a situation-producing theory include goal content, prescriptions for activity, and a survey list outlining the particulars of a situation. In their work, these theorists sought to articulate all of the knowledge required for practice. It is interesting to note that they did not address the realm of manual or technical skill.

As a result of her analysis of the nature of practice theory, Beckstrand (1978a) concluded that the knowledge required for nursing practice consists solely of scientific knowledge of "change and action" (p. 175), ethics, and logic. Like Dickoff and James, Beckstrand (1978b) conceptualized nursing practice as primarily a rational activity in which objective knowledge is applied to particular situations: "It appears that science and ethics are conceptual systems that may completely fulfill the purpose of practice when used in conjunction with the activity of the practitioner and client" (p. 136). All three authors provide some indication that the skill of the practitioner is a notable ingredient in nursing practice, yet this component or element is left to the background and seems to be of lesser importance or secondary to what is speculative.

Lorraine Walker (1971a, 1971b) also examined the knowledge necessary for nursing practice. She concluded that such knowledge takes two principal forms: principles and procedures. Procedures, as conceived by Walker, designate the concrete steps to be taken to bring about a state of affairs. Principles, on the other hand, are more general and take one of four forms: prudential rules, therapeutic rules, ideological rules, and logistics. Walker argued that the practical knowings of nursing are not disciplinary in nature because they are not of a generalizable form, in that they do not apply to every situation, nor are they logically organized. Walker concluded that disciplinary or generalizable knowledge does not directly guide nursing practice.

Barbara Carper (1975, 1978) noted that many contemporary theorists have emphasized the objective, scientific knowledge necessary for nursing practice, to the exclusion of other kinds of knowledge. She opined: "One is almost led to believe that the only valid and reliable knowledge is that which is empirical, factual, objectively descriptive, and general. There seems to be a self-conscious reluctance to extend the term knowledge to include those aspects of knowing in nursing that are not the result of empirical investigation" (1975, pp. 147-148). Carper concluded that there are four domains of knowledge required for nursing practice: empirics, aesthetics, personal knowledge, and ethics. Her work was pivotal in that she expanded the emerging view regarding the knowledge necessary for nursing practice to include more subjective ways of knowing, such as personal knowledge and aesthetics. According to Carper, both forms of knowing are subjective, nondiscursive, and refer to the private insights grounded in the unique experiences and perceptions of the nurse.

Parse's (1981) description of the knowledge required for nursing practice is unique in that she rejects the notion that nursing is guided by prescriptions and rules and maintains that nursing practice is guided by a form of "human science." According to Parse, this knowledge is speculative in nature and describes the meaning of experiences as they are lived. She maintains that nurses use these meanings and insights as they engage and interact with their clients. Although she posits that these principles of human science are objective, in that they are verifiable and sharable, it is unclear how nurses use these principles to guide their practice.

In recent years, several nurses have explored the personal knowledge used in nursing practice. Benner's work is noteworthy in that she suggests that the knowledge necessary for nursing practice is embedded in the decisions made by expert nurses in their day-to-day practices, and that not all of this knowledge can be captured in theoretical propositions or, indeed, identified (Benner, 1983). Based on interviews with expert nurses, Benner has attempted to "articulate" this embedded knowledge. She argues that the process of making an expert judgment in clinical practice is not based on objective knowledge, but on the intuitive judgments of the nurse. Nursing intuition, or having a feel or sense of what should be done, is acquired through experience (Benner & Tanner, 1987). For example, Benner, Tanner, and Chesla (1992) maintain that, rather than using a reasoning process, the expert directly apprehends the action required in a situation. Much of this knowledge is embodied in that it is rapid and nonreflective, is possessed bodily as a habit or skill, and relies on bodily senses. Benner and her colleagues conclude that the major source of knowledge used in expert practice is gained via experience; theory or generalizable knowledge remains in the background, and is used by nurses only when they are unsure about how to proceed.

Beyond possessing expert knowledge about what should be done, Benner (1991) contends that, through experience, nurses develop an understanding of what is respectful or appropriate in particular situations. Benner refers to this knowledge as "skillful ethical comportment" and says that it is a way of knowing that develops over time through experience. Rather than basing decisions on ethical principles or rules, nurses learn to "sense" what is good and not good in various situations.

The advent of what has come to be known as postmodernism and a growing concern and skepticism about the current technological era have prompted many nursing scholars to doubt the place of objective knowledge in nursing practice (indeed, many doubt if objective knowledge of any kind is possible) (see Dzurec, 1995; Henderson, 1995). Nursing scholars such as Bishop and Scudder (1990) and Gadow (1990) have turned their attention almost exclusively to the realm of the subjective or personal. Gadow (1990) maintains that the notion of "objective" knowledge is flawed in that all knowledge is contextual and personal, because we cannot disengage from our subjectivity. She contends that the knowledge required for nursing practice is subjective, and that the central mission of nursing, caring, more than any other human activity, entails subjectivity. Similarly, Bishop and Scudder (1990) contend that nursing practice is a kind of "extrascientific praxis," and that, rather than nurses' applying objective knowledge to practical situations, the practical knowledge of nursing accrues over time within the context of practice. What unites these scholars' positions is their rejection of the objective and their location of the knowledge required for nursing practice within the subjective realm.

AN EXAMINATION OF SELECTED CONCEPTUALIZATIONS

In examining the selected conceptualizations of the knowledge necessary for nursing practice, certain trends in thinking are apparent. We have created a simple classification by contrasting these conceptualizations in relation to two dimensions (objective versus subjective and practical versus speculative) (see Figure 1.1). For example, one domain, Quadrant A, includes knowledge that is both practical and objective. Examples of such knowledge include Nightingale's rules, Dickoff and James's situation-producing theory, the ethics and logic referred to by Beckstrand, and Walker's principles and procedures for nursing practice. A second quadrant, Quadrant B, is both subjective and practical and consists of practical insights and wisdom. Such knowledge may include nurses' ethical and skillful comportment as described by Benner, Carper's aesthetic and personal knowledge, the experiential knowledge referred to by Nightingale, and the manual skill referred to by Stewart. A third quadrant, Quadrant C, includes knowledge that is both objective and speculative. Examples of this kind of knowledge include the natural sciences of anatomy and biology (e.g., Nightingale), the human sciences of Parse (1981), and nursing science (e.g., Carper, Stewart, and Goodrich). Finally, a fourth quadrant, Quadrant D, includes knowledge that is both subjective and speculative. Whereas practical subjective knowledge concerns insights about what should be done, speculative subjective knowledge concerns insights about that which is the case and is descriptive in nature. Examples of this knowledge include intuition, particularly pattern recognition (e.g., Benner), and a component of Carper's aesthetics in which meaning is grasped.

Over time, the importance placed on any one quadrant has shifted. Beginning with Nightingale, we see a primary focus on Quadrant B, practical and subjective knowledge. Stewart and Goodrich called for a greater balance between Quadrants C and B as nursing science emerged. With the emergence of concern about the professionalization of nursing and the development of nursing knowledge came a concomitant devaluing of the realm of nursing that included experience and skill. The debate that emerged from the work of Dickoff, James, Beckstrand, and Walker focused, for the most part, on the nature of the objective realms, both the speculative and the practical. Carper provided a new view on the question regarding the knowledge necessary for nursing practice by arguing that nursing practice requires many ways of knowing, including objective and subjective forms of knowledge. Most recently, the tide has turned and much of nursing's attention has been directed toward the subjective realm. Although one

	Objective Knowledge	Subjective Knowledge
Practical Knowledge	Nursing Rules, Principles, and Procedures Ethical Principles Situation-Producing Theory Logic Practical Nursing Science A	B Practical Wisdom (insights about what should be done) Prudence Clinical Judgment Ethical Comportment Manual Skill Body Knowledge Aesthetics (creative intuition)
Speculative Knowledge	C Natural Science (descriptive, explanatory, including anatomy, biology) Human Sciences Empirics Nursing Science	D Intuition (insight about what is happening) Pattern Recognition Aesthetics Personal Knowledge

Figure 1.1. Possible Conceptualizations of the Knowledge Used in Nursing Practice

might want to conclude that we have come full circle in that we seem to be emphasizing, once again, the kinds of knowledge contained in Quadrant B, there are vast differences. Although Nightingale emphasized the experiential, she also recognized that objective rules and the natural sciences contribute, in a vital way, to nursing practice. In the current era, many theorists appear to focus exclusively on the subjective realm.

The classification we have provided is simple and, to many, may seem procrustean. Clearly, finer distinctions can be drawn between nursing theorists' various positions. We are not suggesting that the domains of knowledge described in our classification provide an adequate description of the knowledge necessary for nursing practice, or that all are essential. We intend this classification only as a heuristic device for uncovering trends in conceptualizations and for pointing to some pertinent distinctions. Inherent in the aforementioned conceptualizations of the knowledge used in nursing practice are several important epistemological questions. Some of these concern the distinctions made in the classification itself. For example, is practical nursing knowledge different from speculative nursing knowledge? Are there different kinds of practical nursing knowledge? Other questions that arise include, How is the knowledge used in nursing practice developed? How is it used? Having set the stage by describing various conceptualizations, we turn our attention to an exploration of possible answers to these questions.

Is Practical Nursing Knowledge Different From Speculative Nursing Knowledge?

As we have described it above, practical knowledge is often described in opposition to speculative knowledge. Wallace (1983), for example, argues that practical knowledge is causative of things, whereas speculative knowledge is merely apprehensive of them. This dichotomy is present in various forms in the nursing literature. In exploring this dichotomy, we ask, Is this distinction appropriate? And on what basis is it made?

The categorical distinction between speculative and practical knowledge may be analytically sound because, through a process of analysis, we can discern characteristics that set these two forms of knowledge apart. First, these forms of knowledge serve different goals or ends. Speculative knowledge is directed toward knowing for the sake of knowing, whereas practical knowledge is directed toward knowing for the sake of doing or making. Second, because their goals differ, speculative knowledge and practical knowledge are concerned with different matters. Speculative knowledge is concerned with things that we can know, not with what we can do. Practical knowledge, on the other hand, is concerned with how we can bring certain things about, what Wallace (1983) refers to as "operables." Additionally, practical knowledge, unlike speculative knowledge, bears on a particular time and a particular operation, and terminates in a specific action. Finally, as we can infer from Audi's (1991) work, speculative knowledge is addressed to us as knowers and practical knowledge, because it concerns what we are to do, is addressed to us as agents.

Although analytically sound, the distinction between the speculative and practical realms appears to disregard the complexity of the relationship between practical and speculative knowledge. Wallace (1983) points out that there are degrees of speculative and practical knowledge. For example, we can have speculative knowledge of something performable or doable. Rather than the two kinds of knowledge being in distinct opposition, there may be a continuum of knowledge, with one end anchored in the speculative realm and the other in the practical. Support for this claim can be located in the work of Maritain (1959), who maintains that there are gradations between practical and speculative knowledge. Maritain posits that as one's proximity to action increases, the nature of the knowledge one requires to act changes. He differentiates among three realms of knowledge: (a) speculative knowledge, which provides theoretic or descriptive explanations; (b) speculatively practical knowledge, which provides theoretic descriptions of things to be done; and (c) practically practical knowledge, which consists of rules for effective action. According to Maritain, practically practical knowledge is more particularized and involves the consideration of the details of a particular case. In the process of determining the kind of action required in a particular case, an individual employs both analytic and composite processes. Maritain's work suggests that the putative dichotomy between the speculative and practical realms inadequately accounts for the knowledge that may underlie any given practice.

Although distinctions can be made between speculative and practical knowledge (including a simple binary distinction and a more complicated gradient), these forms of knowledge are unified in that the intellect that uses them is one and the same. Further, while an individual is making or doing, it is often necessary for him or her to analyze the situation to determine the factors that are at play; hence we use speculative knowledge when acting (see Sarvimäki, 1995). For example, in deciding how best to teach a client about mobilization, we may first analyze the factors that promote or hamper the learning process. We do not stop to ponder whether we are using practical or speculative knowledge as we work through a problem. We move fluidly from analysis to action and back to analysis. Even in the most practical situation, we can theorize. Thus the realms of speculative and practical knowledge may be existentially inseparable, in that they are experienced in unity.

This issue may seem to be more rhetorical than substantial. However, we maintain that our understanding of how the knowledge necessary for nursing practice is best developed must be based on solid epistemic underpinnings. If it is indeed the case that there is an analytic distinction to be made between the practical and speculative realms, and no existential distinction, then we would entreat nursing scholars addressing the topic of the knowledge necessary for nursing practice to indicate clearly whether they are referring to the analytic (ontological) or the existential realm. This is necessary because the conclusions one draws about this knowledge may differ if one is considering the nature of the knowledge rather than questions of how the knowledge is used, applied, and processed. For example, the distinction made by scholars such as Benner (1984), who assert that there are two types of knowledge, "know-how" knowledge and "know-that" knowledge, may be analytically valid but not necessarily existentially valid in nursing practice. Without any epistemic benchmarks to contextualize the claim that there are two types of knowledge, it is difficult to make judgments about its validity.

Are There Different Kinds of Practical Nursing Knowledge?

One difficulty in the discussion of practical nursing knowledge is that it is often assumed that this knowledge is indivisible, in that all forms of practical knowledge are the same. Rather than making this assumption, we ask whether there are importantly different kinds of practical knowledge. A first candidate for consideration, suggested by our classification, is the claim that there are objective and subjective forms of practical knowledge. Audi (1991) has considered the question of whether practical knowledge is objective in the sense of being applicable to anyone and everyone or subjective in that it is applicable only to particular persons in particular situations. The distinction implied by Audi, in our view, is problematic, because he equates objectivity with applicability. We can all imagine exceptional situations in which objective principles do not apply to individual cases. Yet this limitation to the universality of objective principles does not necessarily relegate them to the subjective realm. It may still be the case that there are both subjective and objective forms of practical knowledge.

We contend that the subjective and objective represent two distinct forms of practical nursing knowledge. Subjective practical nursing knowledge consists of the personal intuitions and insights that nurses gain about how to proceed in particular situations. This form of knowledge is subjective in that it cannot be made explicit and is concrete rather than abstract. Objective practical nursing knowledge, on the other hand, consisting of principles of operation, procedures for action, and intervention strategies, is abstract, easily articulated, and thus sharable, and is applied to situations in general rather than particular situations. We contend that both these kinds of practical nursing knowledge are used in nursing practice. This distinction, not often made in the nursing literature, suggests that the criteria for developing, fostering, and evaluating practical nursing knowledge may differ depending on the specific type being considered.

Another distinction to be considered within the realm of practical nursing knowledge is whether there are conscious and unconscious forms of knowledge used in practice. By *unconscious* we mean that the knowledge is possessed and used without mindful reflection or thought. Smith (1988) suggests that there are different levels of cognition used within practice. The lower levels of cognitive human behavior are unconscious and may be thought of as adaptive responses. This kind of knowledge, described by Merleau-Ponty (1942/1963) as *bodily knowledge,* includes such "practices" as walking, running, and speaking. In the case of nursing, this knowledge may include such things as giving an intramuscular injection, washing one's hands, and keeping one's gloved hands above the waist in a sterile environment. These sorts of behavior patterns, according to Merleau-Ponty, become "part of one's flesh" and occur without any conscious recognition. Seemingly higher forms of human cognition are used in such behavior as pattern recognition, in which one's focal awareness is trained to pick up on particular cues. Although one might be trained initially to recognize patterns using particular rules, the rules eventually become unnecessary. What may be a still higher form of cognition involves the complex and conscious decision-making processes that individuals engage in when they are confronted by complex problems and must use theories, principles, and rules as tools.

Within the past two decades, there has been a growing interest among scholars concerning intuitive and seemingly unconscious cognitive processes in nursing decision making (e.g., Benner, 1984; Chinn & Kramer, 1991; Rew, 1988). The work of Polanyi (1962) is often cited to explicate how these tacit or seemingly unconscious processes operate. Although Polanyi's work offers interesting insights and is clearly applicable to certain kinds of situations (e.g., recognizing faces and riding bicycles), it does not adequately address how individuals make decisions in complex situations. Smith's (1988) claim that there are different levels of cognition used within practice is instructive in that it suggests that reliance on only one form of cognition may be inadequate in nursing practice. In light of this, claims that expert nursing practice is characterized solely by intuitive, holistic, cognitive processes require further consideration.

Another related distinction made in the nursing literature is that between discursive and nondiscursive forms of practical nursing knowledge (e.g., Carper, 1975, 1978). By *nondiscursive,* we mean things that are known and cannot be shared because they cannot be articulated. Those forms of knowledge that are unconscious or bodily are clearly nondiscursive. Other forms of knowledge used in practice, such as those used in the process of problem solving, are clearly discursive (we can give reasons for our conclusions and hence our actions). Other forms of knowledge, although often used in an unconscious manner, can be articulated when necessary. For example, although nurses can recognize that a patient is in shock without using any conscious form of reasoning, they can, if asked, describe what they have observed that led to that conclusion. The foregoing discussion demonstrates that the nature of practical knowledge is extremely complex. We suggest that practical nursing knowledge, rather than being homogeneous and indivisible, is a genus with many species.

How Is the Knowledge Used in Nursing Practice Developed?

Several positions are evident in the literature regarding the origins of the knowledge used in nursing practice. For example, some scholars claim that the knowledge used in nursing practice is disciplinary in nature in that it is derived from public inquiry in which a variety of scientific and philosophical methods are used. In other words, they assert that this knowledge is objective in that it can be shared with others and relates to more than only particular cases. Alternatively, some authors claim that the knowledge used in nursing practice is subjective, contextually bound, and developed through experience within the context of nursing situations.

That knowledge is derived from practice is not an untenable assertion. Ryle (1949/1988) argues that "efficient practice precedes the theory of it" (p. 31). This is the case, Ryle maintains, because we develop maxims or theories about practices by observing what works and what does not. Hence one may be able to perform intelligently without knowing the principles underlying one's actions. This seems to be an apt description of Benner's (1984) expert nurses, who "knew" what to do, but apparently could not articulate the reasons for their actions. Benner (1983) writes, "Knowledge development in an applied discipline consists of extending practical knowledge (know-how) through theory-based scientific investigations and through the charting of the existent know-how that develops through the practice of that discipline" (p. 37).

It is likely that some knowledge necessary for nursing practice is developed solely through experience. However, is all knowledge necessary for nursing practice developed in this way? Ryle's (1949/1988) arguments seem to be descriptive of certain kinds of practices, but do they apply to all forms of practice? For some practices it seems evident that it is by thinking about the doing that we theorize about what is taking place. However, this may not work for all practices. It may be the case that an idea about how to act is generated from an individual's experience in practice. The individual must then explore the idea to determine how it can be perfected in practice. This is, we believe, an especially illuminating point, for if it is the case that the knowledge required for practice is derived solely from practice, then all possibilities and potentialities of practice are restricted by what is currently done (Benne, Chin, & Bennis, 1976). Undoubtedly, practitioners, particularly expert practitioners, possess knowledge that goes beyond detached observation and theorizing. Yet it is through detached observation and theorizing that we can fully exploit new possibilities in practice. Newly invented concepts and processes in basic research frequently lead to concepts with practical utility.

How Is Knowledge Used in Practice?

We close this section with a consideration of the existential question, How is knowledge used in nursing practice? An examination of the nursing literature reveals that, for some theorists, knowledge use is conceived as a rational process in which knowledge, facts, and rules are used or applied in a deliberate manner to solve particular problems (e.g., Beckstrand, Dickoff & James). In contrast, others have focused almost exclusively on nonrational, perceptual, and intuitive processes (e.g., Benner, Gadow).

The former position presupposes that reason plays an essential role in the attainment of nursing ends. What it fails to recognize, however, is that practices are not necessarily motivated by rational processes alone. What motivates people to act? Some may answer "rationality," but other things motivate individuals to act as well. Greenspan (1988), for example, points out that emotions may function as justifications for action and maintains that feeling states may be just as warranted as rational states. Further, emotion may supplement rational processes by adding further, and perhaps immediate, motivation to act. Rather than viewing the use of knowledge as either intuitive (perceptual) or rational, we suggest that both processes are an integral part of knowledge use.

Another remaining question concerns how speculative insights inform nursing practice. The problem of deriving direction for action from a statement of what is the case seems to create an insurmountable barrier between propositional statements and action—one cannot logically derive an "ought" from an "is" statement. Yet insights and meaning gained from speculative knowledge can influence behavior. Van Manen (1990) points out that an understanding of human experience can help an individual to gain insights that he or she might otherwise lack. Such insights, or enhanced awareness of human experience, are likely to bring practitioners closer to "decisively acting in . . . situations that ask for such action" (p. 154). Additionally, such insights can help to shape the tone of an interaction. Speculative knowledge of human experience can stimulate "tactful thoughtfulness" on the part of practitioners, particularly in relation to their clients. This explanation seems to create new possibilities for the resolution of the intractable problem of how speculative knowledge bears on practical problems and is worthy of further consideration.

SUMMARY AND CONCLUSIONS

We have explored the nature of the knowledge used in nursing practice by providing a brief overview of various conceptualizations of this knowledge, how they have developed historically, and by considering several issues that emerge from such conceptualizations. Our analysis has been limited in that we have not considered every aspect of the knowledge used in practice. Nor have we analyzed all of the writings relevant to the topic. We have attempted to obviate those issues that we believe to be most pressing and yet, for the most part, remain unexplored within the nursing literature. However, in so doing, we have failed to tackle any one issue in sufficient depth. By highlighting the issues, we hope to motivate closer examination of the nature of the knowledge used in nursing practice.

The central proposition that can be drawn from this analysis is that the knowledge used in nursing practice is multifarious and must be considered from the standpoint of its nature (its ontology) and its use. Our initial analysis points to two possible dimensions along which this knowledge can be classified. These include the categorizations of objective versus subjective and speculative versus practical. Other dimensions are suggested by the consideration of the nature of practical nursing knowledge (i.e., discursive versus nondiscursive and conscious versus unconscious). These dimensions represent the possible complexities inherent in the knowledge used in nursing practice.

NOTES

1. We focus our discussion on select knowledge that is used in nursing practice by nurses. We do not address the "commonsense knowledge," held by nurses and other people, that is necessary but not specific to nursing. Such knowledge consists of everyday beliefs, facts, and practices about the world that are generally held and taken for granted, such as the belief that there is a material world and that other human beings, besides ourselves, exist. Additional, although perhaps more mundane, examples include knowledge of how to open doors, knowledge of what various colors are called, and the ability to recognize others.

2. It should be noted that we have not limited the term *knowledge* to refer to that which is strictly discursive or cognitive. Our reference is fairly wide and includes such realms as the moral, the personal, and art as well as science and philosophy (Phenix, 1964). Accordingly, the definition we provide is not sufficiently stringent to meet the requirements of disciplinary knowledge. Based on the work of Kikuchi (1992) and Adler (1965), we assert that disciplinary knowledge is testable by reference to evidence, subject to rational criticism, rectifiable, and falsifiable. Knowledge used in practice, particularly knowledge that is personal or subjective, although essential, falls outside the nursing discipline (we equate the nursing discipline with nursing's body of knowledge) and, therefore, need not be subject to the same exacting criteria. We do not equate that knowledge used by practitioners with the nursing discipline; the latter is part of the former. Nurses use all kinds of knowledge, much of which is not disciplinary.

3. Although many distinguish theoretical knowledge from practical knowledge, we have elected to use the term *speculative knowledge* rather than *theoretical knowledge*. We made this decision because the term *theoretical* is "loaded," in that many definitions of it exist and, particularly within the present context, it is fraught with ambiguity.

REFERENCES

Adler, M. J. (1965). *The conditions of philosophy*. New York: Atheneum.

Angeles, P. A. (1981). *Dictionary of philosophy*. New York: Barnes & Noble.

Audi, R. (1991). *Practical reasoning*. London: Routledge.

Beckstrand, J. (1978a). The need for a practice theory as indicated by the knowledge used in the conduct of practice. *Research in Nursing and Health, 1*, 175-179.

Beckstrand, J. (1978b). The notion of a practice theory and the relationship of scientific and ethical knowledge to practice. *Research in Nursing and Health, 1*, 131-136.

Benne, K. D., Chin, R., & Bennis, W. G. (1976). Science and practice. In W. G. Bennis, K. D. Benne, R. Chin, & K. E. Corey (Eds.), *The planning of change* (3rd ed., pp. 128-137). New York: Holt, Rinehart & Winston.

Benner, P. (1983). Uncovering the knowledge embedded in clinical practice. *Image: The Journal of Nursing Scholarship, 15,* 36-41.

Benner, P. (1984). *From novice to expert: Excellence and power in clinical nursing practice.* Menlo Park, CA: Addison-Wesley.

Benner, P. (1991). The role of experience, narrative, and community in skilled ethical comportment. *Advances in Nursing Science, 14*(2), 1-21.

Benner, P., & Tanner, C. (1987). Clinical judgment: How expert nurses use intuition. *American Journal of Nursing, 87,* 23-31.

Benner, P., Tanner, C., & Chesla, C. (1992). From beginner to expert: Gaining a differentiated clinical world in critical care nursing. *Advances in Nursing Science, 14*(3), 13-28.

Bishop, A. H., & Scudder, J. R., Jr. (1990). *The practical, moral, and personal sense of nursing: A phenomenological philosophy of practice.* Albany: State University of New York Press.

Carper, B. A. (1975). Fundamental patterns of knowing in nursing. *Dissertation Abstracts International, 36*(10), 4941B. (University Microfilms No. AAC76-7772)

Carper, B. A. (1978). Fundamental patterns of knowing in nursing. *Advances in Nursing Science, 1*(1), 13-23.

Chinn, P. L., & Kramer, M. K. (1991). *Theory and nursing: A systematic approach* (3rd ed.). St. Louis, MO: Mosby-Year Book.

Dickoff, J., & James, P. (1968). A theory of theories: A position paper. *Nursing Research, 17,* 197-203.

Dzurec, L. C. (1995). Poststructuralist science: An historical account of profound visibility. In A. Omery, C. E. Kasper, & G. G. Page (Eds.), *In search of nursing science* (pp. 233-244). Thousand Oaks, CA: Sage.

Gadow, S. (1990). The advocacy covenant: Care as clinical subjectivity. In S. Stevenson & T. Tripp-Reimer (Eds.), *Knowledge about care and caring: State of the art and future development. Proceedings of a Wingspread Conference.* Kansas City, MO: American Academy of Nursing.

Goodrich, A. W. (1912). The complete nurse. *American Journal of Nursing, 12,* 777-782.

Greenspan, P. S. (1988). *Emotions and reasons: An inquiry into emotional justification.* New York: Routledge.

Henderson, D. J. (1995). Consciousness raising in participatory research: Method and methodology for emancipatory nursing inquiry. *Advances in Nursing Science, 17*(3), 58-69.

Kikuchi, J. F. (1992). Nursing questions that science cannot answer. In J. F. Kikuchi & H. Simmons (Eds.), *Philosophic inquiry in nursing* (pp. 26-37). Newbury Park, CA: Sage.

Maritain, J. (1959). *The degrees of knowledge* (G. B. Phelan, Trans.). New York: Charles Scribner's Sons.

Merleau-Ponty, M. (1963). *The structure of behavior* (A. L. Fisher, Trans.). Boston: Beacon. (Original work published 1942)

Montag, M. L. (1951). *The education of nursing technicians.* New York: G. P. Putnam's Sons.

Nightingale, F. (c. 1899). *Training of nurses and nursing the sick.* London: Spottiswoode. (Microfiche: Adelaide Nutting Historical Nursing Collection)

Nightingale, F. (1969). *Notes on nursing: What it is, and what it is not.* New York: Dover. (Original work published 1860)

Palmer, I. S. (1983). Nightingale revisited. *Nursing Outlook, 31,* 229-233.

Parse, R. R. (1981). *Man-living-health: A theory of nursing.* Albany, NY: Delmar.

Phenix, P. H. (1964). *Realms of meaning: A philosophy of the curriculum for general education.* New York: McGraw-Hill.

Polanyi, M. (1962). Tacit knowing: Its bearing on some problems of philosophy. *Reviews of Modern Physics, 34,* 601-616.

Rew, L. (1988). Nurses' intuition. *Applied Nursing Research, 1,* 27-31.

Rogers, M. E. (1961). *Educational revolution in nursing.* New York: Macmillan.

Ryle, G. (1988). *The concept of mind.* London: Penguin Group. (Original work published 1949)

Sarvimäki, A. (1995). *Knowledge in interactive practice disciplines: An analysis of knowledge in education and health care.* Stockholm: Stockholm University College of Health Sciences, Unit for Research and Development.

Smith, B. (1988). Knowing how vs. knowing that. In J. C. Nyíri & B. Smith (Eds.), *Practical knowledge: Outlines of a theory of traditions and skills* (pp. 1-16). London: Croom Helm.

Stewart, I. M. (1922). The evolution of nursing education. *American Journal of Nursing, 22,* 329-334.

Stewart, I. M., Clayton, L. S., & Jamme, A. C. (1916). The aims of the training school for nurses. *American Journal of Nursing, 16,* 319-328.

van Manen, M. (1990). *Researching lived experience: Human science for an action sensitive pedagogy.* London, ON: Althouse.

Walker, L. O. (1971a). Nursing as a discipline. *Dissertation Abstracts International, 32*(06), 3459B. (University Microfilms No. AAC72-1528)

Walker, L. O. (1971b). Toward a clearer understanding of the concept of nursing theory. *Nursing Research, 20,* 428-435.

Wallace, W. A. (1983). *From a realist point of view.* Lanham, MD: University Press of America.

Knowing the Patient?

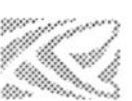

JOAN LIASCHENKO

Recent research has emphasized that "knowing the patient" is a critical aspect of nursing practice (Fisher, Fonteyn, & Liaschenko, 1994; Jenny & Logan, 1992; Liaschenko, 1993; Tanner, Benner, Chesla, & Gordon, 1993). Social practices deal in some way with human beings, and how human beings are understood varies in keeping with those practices. In everyday nursing language, *patients* and *persons* are terms used to refer to the individual human beings for whom nurses care. Indeed, it seems that these categories are used interchangeably, although *patient* is certainly the more common term. Reflecting the practice they studied, the investigators cited above also use both terms, and yet what they mean by *knowing the patient* varies both across and within the research. So we might wonder, What's in a name? Within the context of this work, part of the answer is knowledge. *Knowing the patient* and *knowing the person* refer to

---

AUTHOR'S NOTE: This research was supported through a National Research Service Award Predoctoral Fellowship (F31 NR06836) from the National Institute for Nursing Research, a PEO Scholar's Award, a University of California Graduate Research Award, and a UCSF School of Nursing Century Club Research Award. I would like to thank Mr. Jim Eilers, Anastasia Fisher, RN, DNSc, and Sara Weiss, RN, PhD, for their helpful comments during the preparation of this chapter.

decidedly different kinds of knowledge. In addition to knowledge of the patient and the person, nursing practice requires knowledge of the case. This chapter is a beginning attempt to clarify these different knowledges and to examine where they are separate and where they overlap. Specifically, I am concerned with understanding what it means for a nurse to know a patient as a person. What kind of knowledge is person knowing, and what relevance does this hold for the work of nursing? *Meaning* may have symbolic, normative, and empirical associations (Jaggar, 1991); I use *meaning* here to refer to the empirical associations of knowing the person within the context of nursing practice. This chapter is developed from a study of nurses for whom knowing the patient as person is to know something about what it is for the patient to have a life (Liaschenko, 1993).

THE INDIVIDUAL, NURSING, AND DIFFERENT TYPES OF KNOWLEDGE

When a nurse makes the claim that she or he knows a patient, what is it that she or he knows and how is this knowledge accessed? In our research, my colleagues and I have found that nurses know individuals as cases, as patients, and as persons (Fisher et al., 1994). While my colleagues did ethnographic fieldwork in a psychiatric emergency service and a cardiovascular and neurological intensive care unit (ICU), I conducted a narrative study of home care and psychiatric nurses, using unstructured interviews. Although knowing the patient was central and common to all of our research, we came to see through our discussions that *knowing the patient* was used by nurses to refer to different types of knowledge, types that we labeled *case, patient,* and *person.* These terms reflect, in part, the ways in which the physical body of the patient is located in space and time in relation to the work of nursing and in the landscape of contemporary health care structures.

The Case: The "Disembodied" Patient

What kind of knowledge is knowledge of the case? It is mostly biomedical, but not exclusively. Case knowledge is the generalized knowledge of physiology, diagnosis, treatment possibilities, and statistical outcomes. No particular physical body, nor indeed any body, is required for a nurse to have case knowledge. Knowing the case is an example par excellence of what Arney and Bergen (1984) call the "disappearance of the experiencing patient" (p. 8). The ontological entity dissolves under the scrutiny of the medical gaze and is reduced to that part in need of fixing. In the situation of the case, the individual is a passive object on which a nurse acts. Access to knowledge is limited to objectified physiological and psychological data, and the relationship between person and nurse focuses on the functioning and monitoring of physical and psychological processes. Moral responsibility on the nurse's part lies in attending to the precarious physiological status of the person, with the goal of establishing stability.

In their work, Fisher and Fonteyn illustrated how knowledge of the individual is structured by physical design and the organization of work. Not only are ICUs designed to facilitate probing and monitoring of every physiological process, but many of them, at least in tertiary facilities, are designed to serve those with one classification of physiological dysfunction and/or one set of procedures or interventions. For example, Fisher and Fonteyn conducted fieldwork in ICUs that care only for postoperative open heart surgery or neurosurgical cases. The individuals who undergo such treatments are, for the most part, in these places for exceedingly short periods of time, and are sometimes barely conscious. For the nurses in the ICUs Fisher and Fonteyn studied, aspects of "knowing the case" included knowing the physicians, surgery, physiology, protocols, indicators and range of patient outcomes, anticipated complications, and usual therapeutic interventions. All of this knowledge is biomedical, with the exception of knowing the physicians, which is a particularized knowing that tells nurses the leeway they have within protocols, when to call physicians, and the physicians' success rates and competence. These latter two set up a pattern of expectations of what might present itself in the clinical situation. For the nurses these researchers studied in the psychiatric emergency service, "knowing the case" included knowledge of the working diagnoses, indicators and range of patient outcomes, general responses to therapy, and typical clinical interventions.

The Patient

Knowledge of the patient requires the particularity of a body. When the generalized knowledge of physiology, pathology, diagnosis, and therapeutics becomes concrete in the body of the sick individual, case knowledge is transformed into patient knowledge. Although particularity is central to Fisher et al. (1994), Jenny and Logan (1992), and Tanner et al. (1993), how these researchers understand it varies.

For Fisher and Fonteyn, "knowing the patient" includes knowledge of the individual's history, demographics (such as age, gender, socioeconomic status, and marital status), and support systems. This is not only knowledge *of* the patient, it creates the patient. These categories endow the particularity that has become concrete in the body with an identity suited to the purposes of health care institutions. "Knowing the person" for these researchers is a matter of understanding the individual's physical and emotional responses to treatment.

Fisher and Fonteyn are precise in their descriptions, making clear distinctions among case, patient, and person knowledge. In contrast, Jenny and Logan (1992) and Tanner et al. (1993) seem to use the terms *patient* and *person* interchangeably, but the knowledge they discuss is essentially that of patient response patterns to interventions. Access to this knowledge is largely through the world of the health care system. When nurses know the patient, they know the individual through the realm of work and routines. In this context, individuals are not passive objects on which nurses act, but neither are they seen as persons with unique histories, with their own desires, intentions, and limits. In one example, however, Tanner et al. (1993) approach the understanding of knowing the person in the way that I will discuss in the remainder of this chapter.

The Person

In contrast to case and patient knowledge, to know an individual as a person is to know her or him as a subject who acts with her or his own desires and intentions. A subject has a personal biography and shares in a collective history (Personal Narratives Group, 1989). When we know a person, we know something about her or his biography or life story. Such an understanding necessarily implies knowing about how the person is situated in and engages with the world.

Whereas Jenny and Logan (1992), Tanner et al. (1993), and my colleagues Fisher and Fonteyn explicitly set out to study clinical knowledge, I did not. I set out to study the ethical concerns of home care and psychiatric nurses. As this research is described elsewhere (Liaschenko, 1993), I need not repeat the description of the project here except to say that I asked study participants to tell me stories from their practice that highlighted some ethical concerns they had about their practice. Part of their answers involved knowing the person, although they frequently used the term *patient.* For these nurses, however, knowing the person was not case knowledge, nor was it the knowledge of individualized responses to therapeutic interventions. It was knowledge of biographical life (Brody, 1987; Bury, 1982), that is, what it meant for the individual to have a specific history and live a particular life.

WHAT IS "KNOWING THE PERSON" KNOWLEDGE OF?

To have a life is to have a sense of agency, to live a temporal and spatial existence and to die (Rachels, 1986). The brief description and the narratives that follow are intended to illustrate these conceptualizations as they were understood by the nurses I interviewed.

Agency

For the nurses in this study, knowing the patient as a person was not merely some instrumental technique to get the patient to do something; rather, it was a deep commitment to patient agency and to the recognition of the life that agency can bring about. Agency is the capacity to initiate meaningful action, and it is through our actions that we craft a life within both social space and temporal parameters. Knowledge of a person is partly a knowledge of how that person lives, as well as what she or he lives for. Disease and illness threaten and sometimes change drastically a person's agency and therefore the kind of life she or he can lead (Charmaz, 1991). For these nurses, protecting and nurturing patient agency is a central moral feature of nursing work. The life must remain the person's life and not become some event in the triumph over disease. Nurses hope that by supporting patients' agency, patients will make decisions and act in ways that make sense in their particular life circumstances. As one psychiatric nurse remarked:

> We're talking about patients' lives, you know. . . . We think we know better than everybody else. We know how you can live your life better. You must measure up to this standard in order to be happy. We've decided this. But there are lots of different ways to be in life, and there's lots of different ways to be happy. And until the point that they're unhappy with their lives and want to move on, that's when it's going to work and that's when I can help them. We can work together to make that better. But that's a shared goal. Otherwise you're trying to live somebody's life for them.

Temporal Dimensions

There are temporal dimensions to having a life. Human beings have a beginning with birth and an ending with death. Between these markers, our lives are structured by temporal patterns. These patterns are physiological rhythms as well as what I call routines of lived experience. By this I mean that the actions through which individuals express their engagement with the world—through their connections to others, to work, to projects and leisure—are temporally structured. This temporality is more than clock time; it contributes to our identity and individuality. When our routines of lived experience are disrupted by disease, injury, or disaster, our subjective sense is that our lives, and not merely patterns of clock time, are affected (Charmaz, 1991). Indeed, it is the disruption of the routines of lived experience that constitutes the experience of illness (Kleinman, 1988). Much of the work of nursing practice is concerned with creating and managing routines of lived experience. We attempt to take the disruption of disease and illness and render it a manageable element integrated into the life experience of the person. The aim of the routines of nursing work is to contribute to the achievement of some state of good for the patient. Nurses help the patient integrate treatment regimens into the pattern of daily life, which is especially important when the disease is chronic. When this is successful, patients can continue to have a sense of confidence about living their lives. Knowledge of the routines of lived experience is knowledge of how people live a temporally structured existence; it is attendance to how the ordering of their lives gives meaning, and it is attendance to the disruptions of those orderings.

> When I go out to see some adults, a lot of what you see with them is the totally other spectrum of life, and how do they feel about being where they are now? So often they're depressed because they're seeing how frail they are and that their bodies aren't working the way they used to work. They're upset and they're frustrated about that. And then there's so many other things that they're angry about—the system doesn't work for them anymore the way it did. Things they took for granted, like driving, [aren't] even an option now. (home care nurse)

Spatial Dimensions

In referring to the spatial dimensions of having a life, I mean that we have bodies and therefore occupy physical, social, and political space. It follows, then, that people as embodied beings must be somewhere—that is, must have a place. Although place can be viewed from several frameworks, the nurses with whom I spoke referred to it in two senses. First, people occupy social space in that they share in the lives of others. Our identity as agents is constituted in interactions with significant others—interactions that occur in certain spaces, thus making the spaces themselves meaningful to us. Our connection to others is made manifest in the spaces we inhabit. Although this need for a sense of belonging somewhere was related by both groups of nurses, home care nurses, because they had formerly practiced in hospitals, were particularly cognizant of the home as indicative of the belongingness of the patient. As one home care nurse indicated, patients' personal geographies can show you their lives:

> I never knew where anybody lived. Everybody is so much more alike in the hospital because they're all in their patient gowns and you don't see what's in their luggage. You don't see the bags that they bring in.

> So there's a lot of stuff that you just really don't see in the hospital that, when you get to see them at home, you see a whole different person. At home you see the other things that they're dealing with, besides whatever made them go into the hospital.

In the second sense of social space, these nurses viewed place in a social and political context, in which different people occupy different social positions, with corresponding access or impediment to social resources, specifically health care. These nurses were especially concerned about poverty and the damage poverty inflicts on what it means to have a life. These issues will be discussed further in another work, but I wanted to make note of them here because they are a major constituent of biographical life and what it means to have a life.

Knowledge of a person's agency and of the temporal and spatial dimensions of her or his existence is biographical knowledge. Such knowledge recognizes that for human beings, agency, time, and space are defining matters; they constitute our identity and define our relationships. What is significant and what is potentially problematic about such knowledge in nursing?

THE SIGNIFICANCE OF KNOWING THE PERSON

The question remains, Why is knowledge of the person important? What is the significance of such knowledge to nursing practice? Nursing is an interventionist discipline; that is, it is aimed at doing something to or for people. Knowing the person becomes critically important when the moral work of nursing practice includes acting for individuals, with the aim of helping them to maintain the integrity of their lives, to take up their lives after disease or injury, and to face progressive deterioration and death (Liaschenko, 1995b). Acting for patients in these ways can require more than case or patient knowledge. Consider the following story:

> I'll start telling you the story. Something happened to me about a year ago. I was seeing a patient, Mrs. A, an older woman, about 75, who lived alone. I'm not sure of her origin but she was European Jewish

> and her family had mostly been decimated in the Holocaust, which was very important in terms of her paranoia and her fears and how that feeds into my actions. She was a diabetic, very brittle, and she'd also had a couple of strokes, which made her memory kind of in and out, and she was really very marginally able to take care of herself. She would show me photo albums, show me little girls that she'd grown up with, and they were all dead. Her sister was dead, her sister's husband, her sister's children were dead, her father was dead, her aunts were—everyone was dead. And she had all these pictures. And she had really been one of the lone survivors. And she was still very alone and still living very much in that world. (home care nurse)

This nurse was called one day by Mrs. A's home health aide, who asked her to come immediately because Mrs. A was grossly confused and disoriented. Her blood glucose was extremely elevated, and the nurse did what immediately needed to be done and then called the physician, who wanted Mrs. A hospitalized. At mention of this, Mrs. A became increasingly agitated, screaming that she would not go and demanding that the nurse leave her house. Several hours went by as the nurse contacted Mrs. A's daughter in a distant city and the daughter decided to come, but this was not immediately helpful. The nurse wanted a psychiatrist to come to the house, but the home care agency was not able to provide one at the time and did not help the nurse explore other psychiatric avenues. Somehow the nurse learned that she could have had Mrs. A committed against her will, but given Mrs. A's background, the nurse did not believe this was a satisfactory solution. The nurse continued:

> She said, "Get out of my house. I want you out of here." And she was starting to clear a little bit more mentally, I guess because her insulin kicked in and she'd had a piece of bread or something. So I really didn't know what to do. She'd say, "I'm asking you to get out of my house. Please get out of my house right now." And, you know, shaking and trying her hardest to concentrate, and all the time kind of weaving like she was going to fall down again. So I really didn't know what to do, because I didn't feel that she was very oriented, and I felt that if the paramedics came and forced her into this ambulance, that it would be sort of like when her family was carted off to the death chambers.

This was a very difficult situation in which the nurse was trying to weigh a variety of factors, including Mrs. A's current physical condition and psychological state and the home care agency's bottom-line policy of safety first, against the woman's history, the integrity that marked her life and constituted her very identity. Here is what the nurse did—and why:

> You know, I'm Catholic and I was born after the war, but it's always been a big part of my personal mythology, if you will. My parents talked about the Holocaust a lot, and I don't know why, but it's just—well, of course it's a very horrifying thing, but it's always seemed very real to me. And just some of the nuts and bolts of it, the children being separated from their parents. If you just think about people taking little children away from their mothers and just the terror, the terror. I hate, I hate to see people in terror. You know this little boy that was kidnapped recently [referring to an incident in the city in which a young child was abducted and killed]? People say, they took his life, he's young, how could they take his life? But all I can think about is the terror of that child between the time he was kidnapped and the time he was dead. So I didn't like to see her terrified. I think that's the horror of it. And that's why I had left, because I—that was the best thing I could think of to do.

This nurse's leaving Mrs. A's home reflects not a simple, linear causality but a final common pathway of action and judgment based on a complex interaction of case, patient, and person knowledges. The disembodied case knowledge of diabetes and its management on which the nurse acted says that a certain blood glucose range is likely to respond to a given amount of insulin.

In remarking that Mrs. A "was starting to clear," the nurse was noting the response to this particular intervention. But her patient knowledge of Mrs. A exceeded this and included, among other factors, that Mrs. A was a brittle diabetic and therefore unstable, that she had multi-infarct dementia, that her daughter would not arrive for several hours, that Mrs. A's capacity to live alone was nearly exhausted, that living with her daughter was not an option, and that Mrs. A was terrified and screaming for the nurse to leave her home.

Providing care in such a situation would be challenging enough without knowledge of Mrs. A as a person. But knowing that Mrs. A lost many members of her family in the Holocaust changed the landscape of the nurse's potential actions. In thinking about what to do, this nurse attended to all knowledges, but it was clearly knowledge of the person that made the greatest claim on her action. She explained her reason for acting in continued dialogue with the interviewer:

Interviewer: It sounds like (and tell me if this is a fair characterization) that, for you, a central ethical grounding of your practice is this issue about terror and what you as a nurse can do to intervene and prevent that.

Nurse: Right. Because I feel that the mental suffering that people have because of their physical problems is the central suffering. And second, I would say, it's the moral precept, if you will, of somebody's right to choose their own fate, even if ostensibly they don't have quite the equipment to do it. No one should be forced to accept medical treatment.

Interviewer: Even if that means it will have a tragic outcome?

Nurse: Sometimes.

The nurse went on to talk about the integrity of the patient's life and, in her view, the refusal of treatment that integrity necessitated. This nurse saw her commitment to the patient as extending beyond the palpable danger of physiological harm to the harm that could result if she were forcibly removed by paramedics because this could reenact that other time, "when her family was carted off to the death chambers." Because this nurse knew Mrs. A as a person, she saw such an intervention on her part as far more dreadful than the risk of further physical harm. This biographical knowledge grounded the nurse's perception of moral salience and provided a reason for her action. Some may not agree that her actions were the "right" ones, *right* referring to what is permissible or sanctioned by custom, law, or some authority. For some, the threat of physical harm or the agency's responsibility for safety might be seen as more significant than the woman's history in relation to the Holocaust. Nonetheless, it can be argued that this nurse did a "good" thing, *good* referring to some desirable state of affairs. For the nurse in this narrative, the good was to try to decrease the woman's terror. Her knowledge of Mrs. A's history provided a reason for the nurse's action and opened up the moral space (Walker, 1993) necessary for understanding and continued dialogue.

Knowing the person requires that one meet the subjectivity of the person with one's own subjectivity. That is, nurses also come to every situation with their own likes, dislikes, moral ideals, and so forth. Their lives, like the lives of patients, are constituted by their agency and routines of lived experience; they occupy a certain social and political space, and they too will die.

SOME IMPLICATIONS OF KNOWING THE PERSON

Although the story related above is dramatic, it is not unusual. Nurses encounter such situations on a regular basis. I believe that knowing the person is important to nursing practice, but it is not without its cautionary side in at least two regards. One concerns its possibility and the other the conditions of its desirability. Regarding possibility, knowing, including knowing a person, is situational; that is, it is determined by the cultural beliefs as well as the temporal and spatial organization by which we create social and moral order. Within health care, some of these spatial, temporal organizations make it impossible for nurses to know the persons they treat in the way I have described. This type of knowledge takes time; it must evolve over the course of numerous interactions. It is not likely that an ICU nurse who works with patients who are being made physiologically stable and who are discharged within days can get to know these persons in this way. In fact, one could argue that any setting in which the primary goal is to control symptoms and move the patient out does not lend itself to knowing the person—and this is precisely the kind of setting that exists in hospitals. Nor is home care immune, as, increasingly, "visits" are being done through telemetry and via telephone as one way to increase productivity and lower costs.

The home care nurse in the above narrative had known this patient over an extended period of time. Should this incident have occurred on a day when this nurse was not there, the covering nurse could not have known Mrs. A as a person in the way I have described. In the absence of such knowledge, the nurse could have acted only on case and patient knowledges. Just to be clear, I am not claiming that the nurse did "the right thing," although I do believe she did a good thing. Certainly there are nurses who would disagree. Nursing has a long history of commitment to the well-being of the individual to which most nurses have been socialized. My point about the idea of possibility, however, is that we may wish to exercise care not to set up expectations that are impossible for nurses to meet. Knowing the person is not always possible. The more complex question is, Even if it were, is it desirable?

Throughout this chapter I have argued that knowing the person is important to nursing; nonetheless, I have reservations about this knowing being seen as an unquestioned good, and I want to raise three issues. The first concerns intrusiveness. If I go to a health care provider for treatment of an ear infection, I might perceive any attention beyond civility and attention to my immediate problem as unnecessary—indeed, as intrusive. I might even imagine that the health care provider is trying to create problems where there are none, problems that are then likely to be deemed fit for intervention by experts. Armstrong (1983) has argued that nurses' increased attention to the subjective experience of the people in their care is evidence of the further surveillance and domination of medicine through the ever-increasing medicalization of our lives. Given that nurses occupy a social space that bears a potentially instrumental relationship to the ends of institutionalized medicine (Liaschenko, 1994, 1995a), Armstrong's point merits serious discussion. As instruments of surveillance, nurses may play an expanding role as the culture, in its current obsession with "healthy lifestyle," holds people increasingly responsible for their health.

The second issue I want to raise regarding the desirability of knowing the person has to do with the implications of such knowing for nurses' actions. Such knowledge does not always simplify, and can even complicate, nursing practice. Attention to the aspects that make a life a particular life is precisely what transforms an individual from a case and a patient to a person. As paradoxical as it may seem, the presence of the person in the patient can muddle the nurse's perception of need and the demand for response that present themselves so potently in the immediacy of the here and now. By this I mean that if the nurse takes into account only those needs that are immediately present through case and patient knowledge, the possibilities for appropriate action are limited, thereby making the responses straightforward. On the other hand, when the nurse perceives these needs against the background of the person's life and values, the ends at which the nurse's actions should be aimed are not always so clear.

There are no a priori meanings in the knowledge of a person. In the example of knowing the person given by Tanner et al. (1993), the meaning of the knowledge of that person's life led to continuing treatment. In the story of Mrs. A, the nurse's knowledge of her life called for the opposite response—to risk her physical danger, even her death, for the sake of an integrity beyond the physical. Being open to the knowledge of what it means for a given person to have a life forces the nurse to acknowledge that there will be times when she or he will disagree with the person. This merits discussion, both among individual nurses and within the discipline. Some of the caring literature seems to contain the message that if nurses simply care enough or in the right ways, individuals' difficulties can be endured, if not transcended. In my mind, there is a subtle but powerful possibility for caring to become coercion in such cases. Knowing Mrs. A as a person was not a rationale for coercion; it was not merely a form of sentimental work (Strauss, Fagerhaugh, Suczek, & Wiener, 1982) enabling the patient to endure some aspect of medical intervention. This narrative brings into sharp relief the fact that nurses sometimes stand as intermediaries, as boundary workers between competing interests and different interpretations of what is good. Acting on the knowledge of what it means for a person to have a life may require that nurses take a stand against received wisdom, be it religious, legal, or medical. Yet to do so is no small matter.

The final issue I want to raise regarding the desirability of knowing the person is that this desirability is political—that is, it is a question for all of society and not merely nursing. Furthermore, the desirability of knowing the person in relevant contexts is a political matter because it addresses the kind of health care we, as a society, envision. In spite of the reservations I have enumerated above, I do believe that knowing the person is important to the care of individuals in some contexts. Earlier, I mentioned that I might regard as intrusive any attempts to know me as a person if I were seeking treatment for an ear infection, a problem I see as temporary and curable. If, however, I were facing a chronic, debilitating, or fatal disease, my life would be interrupted in more than temporary ways (Charmaz, 1991). In such a situation, my ability to have a life and a sense of integrity at all may depend on safe passage through "the kingdom of the sick" (Sontag, 1979, p. 3). A conceptualization of the ends of health care as safe passage challenges the present system's epistemology, wisdom, and allocation of resources. Safe passage involves the kind of knowledge of the person that comes through an attentive gaze and heartfelt listening. Although nurses are not the only ones who are important in this passage, they are unquestionably central. Yet the kind of attentiveness this knowledge demands is increasingly being see as fluff, not essential to a vision of health care in which people are cared for only on the basis of case and patient knowledge. These different types of knowing reflect different commitments to how we want to live. The desirability of knowing the person and the contexts of that knowing are a matter of the kind of world we want to have and the kind of people we want to be.

REFERENCES

Armstrong, D. (1983). The fabrication of nurse-patient relationships. *Social Science and Medicine, 17,* 457-459.

Arney, W. R., & Bergen, B. (1984). *Medicine and the management of living: Taming the last great beast.* Chicago: University of Chicago Press.

Brody, H. (1987). *Stories of sickness.* New Haven, CT: Yale University Press.

Bury, M. (1982). Chronic illness as biographic disruption. *Sociology of Health and Illness, 4,* 167-182.

Charmaz, K. (1991). *Good days, bad days: The self in chronic illness and time.* New Brunswick, NJ: Rutgers University Press.

Fisher, A., Fonteyn, M., & Liaschenko, J. (1994, May). *Knowing: The case, the patient, the person.* Symposium presented at the International Nursing Research Conference, Vancouver.

Jaggar, A. (1991). Feminist ethics: Projects, problems, prospects. In C. Card (Ed.), *Feminist ethics* (pp. 78-104). Lawrence: University Press of Kansas.

Jenny, J., & Logan, J. (1992). Knowing the patient: One aspect of clinical knowledge. *Image: The Journal of Nursing Scholarship, 24,* 254-258.

Kleinman, A. (1988). *The illness narratives: Suffering, healing, and the human condition.* New York: Basic Books.

Liaschenko, J. (1993). *Faithful to the good: Morality and philosophy in nursing practice.* Unpublished doctoral dissertation, University of California, San Francisco.

Liaschenko, J. (1994). The moral geography of home care. *Advances in Nursing Science, 17*(2), 16-26.

Liaschenko, J. (1995a). Artificial personhood: Nursing ethics in a medical world. *Nursing Ethics, 2,* 185-196.

Liaschenko, J. (1995b). Ethics in the work of acting for patients. *Advances in Nursing Science, 18*(2), 1-12.

Personal Narratives Group. (Ed.). (1989). *Interpreting women's lives: Feminist theory and personal narratives.* Bloomington: Indiana University Press.

Rachels, J. (1986). *The end of life: Euthanasia and morality.* Oxford, UK: Oxford University Press.

Sontag, S. (1979). *Illness as metaphor.* New York: Vintage.

Strauss, A., Fagerhaugh, S., Suczek, B., & Wiener, C. (1982). Sentimental work in the technologized hospital. *Sociology of Health and Illness, 4,* 254-278.

Tanner, C., Benner, P., Chesla, C., & Gordon, D. (1993). The phenomenology of knowing the patient. *Image: The Journal of Nursing Scholarship, 25,* 273-280.

Walker, M. (1993). Keeping moral space open: New images of ethics consulting. *Hastings Center Report, 23*(2), 33-40.

Discovering Knowledge in a Practice Setting

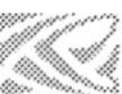

F. NDIDI U. GRIFFIN

When nurses learn about the world of the patient, they can apply that knowledge to a more emancipatory way of being in the practice setting. My purpose in this chapter is to illustrate how I applied the perspectives of patients at a state-operated inner-city clinic to the development of four types of knowledge: structural, communicative, cultural, and social. Throughout the chapter, verbatim comments from patients in this setting serve as a foundation for interpretation of the meanings of these dialogic exchanges and for description of the practice transformations these insights have produced.

STRUCTURAL KNOWLEDGE

Some patients have real concerns regarding the quality of care they receive. For example, regarding such matters as the 10-minute office visit, fees for services, amount of time spent with the caregiver, quality of services rendered, and patient satisfaction, respondents offered varying perspectives. Cynthia perceived the situation as follows:

> One of my problems with health care and the reimbursement mechanism is that if you ask someone to do a job and that person is ordinarily making $10.00 an hour, and you cut your reimbursement down to $3.00 an hour, in my mind that person cuts her service down to $3.00 an hour. So, if I go in with a serious problem, the 10 minutes that the provider would ordinarily give me has already been cut down to 3 minutes because she's got to see two other patients to make her $10.00. So then it cuts down not only on my time, but also on the quality of care I receive.

Rene and Val had the following concerns regarding the 10-minute office visit, patient satisfaction, and the quality of service rendered. Rene said, "I'm afraid to go—they won't take time. I fear they will diagnose the wrong thing." Val noted, "I have a fear of the runaround. They make you not want to go. They don't check you. They don't have you undress. You just feel so small. I would rather be sick, and then I have to go."

On the issue of service satisfaction, Val stated:

> To understand what it feels like being a patient in this clinic, just go through and register, which to me is the demeaning part, and see if you don't feel worse after having seen the provider. If you go because your finger hurts, they talk down to you. Then afterwards, even if your finger has been treated, your whole body has been sort of abused. Mentally and physically you have been abused.

Janet made the following observation regarding the office visit: "Appointments are scheduled around the provider's schedule." In addition, she told of a piecemeal approach used by the provider: "There is segmentation of care. Everyone gets a piece of the action. Stereotyping occurs and an assembly-line approach to care takes over. Basic therapies are not going to work for everybody!"

All four of the women quoted above stated that they would delay entry into the health care system by trying home remedies to cure themselves before seeking care from their providers. Fear of "the runaround," fear of the unknown, fear of inadequate treatment, fear of harm, fear of stereotyping, and fear of a general sense of disrespect were real concerns of these four women.

The comments made by these four patients led me to believe that an examination of the quality of services provided at some of our operating clinics was warranted. Examples of both the piecemeal approach and the assembly-line intake were evident at a Monday-afternoon sexually transmitted disease (STD) clinic. Based on management's expectations, 10-minute patient visits were scheduled. The clinic operation was as follows: A registered nurse would take patients' histories; a family nurse practitioner was responsible for the physical examinations and diagnoses, for furnishing medications, and for instructing the patients on the designated pharmacological and non-pharmacological treatments; a Spanish-speaking interpreter with knowledge of medical terminology and the regional dialect would reinforce instructions in the patients' native language; a technician would collect blood for additional serology and HIV testing if patients' histories warranted these procedures; and, finally, patients would see the STD investigator if their diagnoses demanded locating the patients' sexual contacts for treatment and prevention of the spread of identified diseases. Clearly, fragmentation of care was in full operation at this state-operated clinic. In addition, ethnic, cultural, and gender variations existed. For example, monolingual Spanish-speaking male patients who were accustomed to receiving their care from male providers might find themselves in the care of an English-speaking female.

After becoming aware of the patients' concerns through observation, formal survey, follow-up on reasons for cancellation of appointments, and direct questioning, management made an attempt to alleviate the patients' anxieties by placing a Spanish-speaking male interpreter in both the intake and examination rooms. However, a more efficacious way to meet the needs of this patient population, decrease patient anxiety, and minimize fragmentation of care would have been to hire a bilingual male practitioner who would be responsible for the intake history, physical examination, education, and treatment of this patient population. In addition, an effort was made to lengthen the actual time spent with the provider, from 10 minutes to 20 minutes, by scheduling fewer client visits per hour. It was felt that this additional time would be spent obtaining a comprehensive medical history, delivering information on prevention and anticipatory guidance, and answering questions patients might have regarding their physical and mental health.

Even though the management and health care providers in this clinic meant to do no harm, unknowingly all were part of a disservice to this community. Clearly, nurses care about helping patients. Nevertheless, if nurses do not take the time to solicit information from patients regarding their perceptions of the quality of the care given, it is quite possible that patients' concerns will never be known, and positive changes, in terms of patient well-being and satisfaction with service, might never be realized.

COMMUNICATIVE KNOWLEDGE

Of the many existing problems in clinical settings relating to the nurse-patient dyad, none may be more serious than the problem of ineffective communication. In this day of emphasis on nurse and patient collaboration in the patient's health care and the advent of the use of verbal contracts jointly developed by the nurse and the patient, nurses' knowledge of the communicative styles in the general populations they serve is crucial.

When asked to comment on her experiences in conversation with her health care provider and what she wanted to receive from these exchanges, Cynthia stated that she hoped that "at the end of the dialogue, I would know something—the process would be completed." However, she said, "I waited for several hours and came out at the end of the visit with a return appointment and some pills. I still don't know what was wrong. Ninety percent of healing is knowing what was wrong." As an example of this type of treatment, she offered the following illustration: "If I have this rash because I'm allergic to strawberries and you give me medicine for the rash and don't tell me what caused the rash, I would continue to eat strawberries."

Janet cited lack of effective communication as a barrier to health care, saying, "Health care providers have poor listening skills." She felt that "no one truly assesses for causative factors. I feel I am not given time to talk. It's get your clothes on and see you back in 2 weeks."

Lastly, on the matter of ineffective communication, Val stated, "They don't think they have to explain but you want to hear more. You keep on going and asking questions." Andi added, "Some of it is just words. Providers don't break it down. They talk medical talk. I don't understand."

It should be further noted that all of these patients felt that providers did not ask appropriate questions, nor did they give appropriate answers to the patients' questions. In addition, the patients felt that their providers were annoyed when the patients asked questions. Moreover, these patients felt that the reason their providers did not listen to them was because the providers stereotyped the patients and diagnosed them based on what the providers deemed most likely to be the problem.

Nurses are initiated into the field of nursing in many subtle ways. Recognizing that language is extremely powerful and that the language and culture of the nursing profession are inseparable, adaptation to the verbal and nonverbal communication patterns of the nursing profession plays an important role in the indoctrination and assimilation processes of becoming a professional nurse. Use of the language of nursing and medicine is essential because it indicates solidarity as well as membership in a powerful subculture within the general culture. The benefits of language adaptation are threefold: (a) Its existence is recognized as a force to be contended with by the general society, (b) the power of language is transferred to other manifestations of power within the individual (ego strength can be elevated), and (c) it is a tool used to win the confidence of the general population (Griffin, 1994).

However, medical terminology usage can be a double-edged sword. Although the language of nursing (which I refer to as *nursingese*) denotes a oneness among the nurse, her profession, and other health care professionals, it also can isolate the patient from the health care team. This exclusion can result in semantic confusion, which can be reflected in the assignment of differing meanings to the same words by the nurse and patient, decreased effectiveness of health promotion interventions, and mislabeling of the patient as noncompliant and resistant to proposed change in his or her health status.

Furthermore, a breakdown in communication between the nurse and the patient may occur due to differing perceptions about health and illness and illness management. At this point, implementation of action research, which is conducted to solve a specific, immediate, concrete problem in a local setting (Moore & Burt, 1982), might be of use in identifying the variables in operation in the setting, discovering how these variables might affect the events occurring in the setting, and possibly result in the identification of sound solutions to the problems of miscommunication and patient discontent.

One discovery could be that the nurse may approach the patient in an authoritative and condescending manner, resulting in both an imbalance of power and a fostering of dependency on the part of the patient. In addition, this approach to delivery of care may result in patient dissatisfaction, uncooperativeness, or even refusal of care. The nurse must be aware of these mechanisms at work and attempt to guard against the potential development of professional ethnocentrism.

On the other hand, active listening is demonstrated when the nurse attends to what the patient is saying, at times paraphrasing what the patient has said, asking for patient clarification of the subject matter, and attempting to interpret the language in the context of the environment in which it occurs. Some or all of these techniques could be helpful approaches for nurses to employ when interacting with patients. Such actions not only give patients an opportunity to voice their innermost concerns, but remind the nurse of the power of language and the importance of communicating openly with patients.

CULTURAL KNOWLEDGE

Over an expanse of several hundred years or more, some ethnic minorities in the United States have experienced similarities in their treatment within the dominant population. The philosophy that the true healer knows no race, creed, or color is an ideal and the essence of the nursing arts (Rempusheski, 1989). In nursing education, this ideal has traditionally led instructors to impress upon their students that all patients should be treated the same, regardless of who they are. This view tends to support the concept of a common culture that permits health care providers to perceive all patients as having similar health needs and goals without regard for varying cultural influences.

In actuality, individual health behavior is largely culturally patterned (Tripp-Reimer & Larry, 1989). When patients and health professionals come from different cultures, it is possible that they might hold different health beliefs and expectations for health behaviors, and thus conflicts may result based on differing perceptions of what constitutes appropriate health behavior and health programs (Tripp-Reimer & Larry, 1989).

To illustrate variability in individual patients' perceptions of health, illness, and appropriate treatment modalities, I offer the views of two patient-respondents. Shimada stated:

> Health is a feeling of well-being. It involves all the aspects of life. Illness is the opposite feeling. I don't seek health care immediately. I'm one of those people who usually tries home remedies first. I really think that's because I have some idea of how to care for myself. I will give myself 30 days—using teas and salves. While living in the West Indies, I learned "root" from my mother-in-law. . . . I believe in herbs and things like that. I try those things in advance, and if it doesn't get better, then I'll go to the clinic.

Shimada believes it is important to treat the whole person, or, as she put it, "It is important to treat the mental and physical self." Also, Shimada has a strong belief in "a higher spiritual power" and a spiritual connection with the stars and the earth. She professed, "It is a higher power that keeps us all alive."

Cynthia has a holistic view of health. She perceives the mind, body, and spirit as inseparable:

> Health is a general feeling of well-being—mentally, physically, spiritually—so that not only are there no aches and pains, there's no mental distress or outward pressure. Illness is some sort of disease or problem that disrupts that feeling of well-being. So in my mind, health is the state of well-being and illness is any problem that distorts that state of well-being.

Besides growing and using her own herbs, Cynthia also uses the services of an herbalist. She was able to recall vividly several instances when herbs were used by her parents to treat illness. She has used many of these remedies on her children and grandchildren. During our interactions, Cynthia shared several remedies with me. At times she seemed amazed that I was so uninformed about the use of herbs as curatives for minor illnesses. Later, when I talked with local residents during my travels through the southern United States, I learned that the treatment methods they used were either identical or closely similar to the remedies cited by Cynthia during our clinic conversations.

The marginal status of folk medicine in the United States is reflective of its relationship with modern medicine and its perceived role, among members of mainstream society, in the context of peripheral social formations. Its marginalization is the outcome of a rapport of domination in which it represents the subjugated pole. As a marginal medical ideology, it can be understood both in its inherent organizational structure and in its relations with mainstream ideology (LaGuerre, 1987).

Certain cultural components are present in every ethnic group. Subtle as well as obvious similarities and differences exist among these groups. The dominant culture pattern will be followed by individuals in each culture to varying degrees, perhaps denied by some and not identified but taken for granted by others (White & Parham, 1990). Based on this assumption, in order to advance health care, nurses must gain knowledge of their patients' cultural identities and take them into consideration during all patient contacts.

One way to increase cross-cultural knowledge is to conduct a cultural assessment. A major component of such an assessment is the performance of a systematic appraisal of beliefs, values, and practices in order to determine the context of patient needs and to tailor nursing interventions. In the cultural assessment, the nurse performs a general assessment to obtain an overview of the characteristics of the patient and identifies areas that may potentially require more in-depth assessment. In this assessment, the nurse elicits the client's subjective reasons for seeking care, his or her notions about the problem, and previous and anticipated treatment (Tripp-Reimer & Larry, 1989).

Biases such as likes, dislikes, and stereotypes may be grounded in culture and revealed partially in behaviors. Biases are also revealed in expectations of self and others. Strong moral commitment to a belief may underlie a behavior. Therefore, a multifaceted assessment of culture and ethnicity includes the elicitation of the patient's perceptions of biases and expectations of care. In addition, the health care provider also must examine his or her own biases and expectations of giving and receiving care (Rempusheski, 1989).

Among an array of guidelines suggested in the literature, those put forth by Kupperschmidt (1988) seem to be the most salient for facilitating cross-cultural sensitivity:

1. Frequently, some patients do not distinguish among the physical, mental, psychological, and spiritual aspects of illness, and may bring to each health care situation a mixture of somatic, psychological, and spiritual concerns.
2. Many health beliefs and practices stem from religious ideation, with wide use of religious practices for selected problems; for some, health is frequently viewed as being in balance with nature and with God.
3. For some groups, traditional and folk medicine may be used concurrently for selected illnesses. There may be a general distrust of modern physicians and the curative value of their prescriptions, and hospitals may be viewed as places of death rather than healing.
4. In some groups, an important family or community member must be consulted before an important decision can be made.
5. Physical assessment may require modification of the usual routine. Culturally sensitive nursing care demands that the nurse assess each patient and not assume that a given patient will have typical biogenetic features. Individualized assessment is always important and does not assume a lesser priority for any patient.

During the history and assessment phases of the office visit, the patient is a *cultural informant.* If the nurse can elicit from the patient problem-specific cultural information, this can be extremely useful in the diagnosis and treatment plan phases of the visit. During the treatment plan phase, nurse and patient negotiate the development of a contract they both can live with. In my own experience, many times, following a course of waiting to see if a problem will either resolve without intervention or following a course of home treatment, my patients have presented plans that include incorporation of their own belief systems.

As a result of working in several state-funded clinics, I have grown to appreciate the importance of cultural negotiation. Cultural negotiation, or cultural brokerage, consists of acts of translation in which messages, instructions, and belief systems are manipulated, linked, or processed between the professional and the lay models of health problems and preferred treatment. In each, attention is given to eliciting the patient's views regarding the illness experience (Kupperschmidt, 1988). Subsequently, attention is given to providing scientific information while acknowledging that the patient may hold different views.

Medical science has gathered scientific knowledge about the etiology of many disease processes. However, medical practitioners must remember that the client's perception of the health problem, its cause, and possible treatment is a crucial element for the design of a long-lasting behavior change project. Patients' traditional ethnic backgrounds may lead them to use warm sweet oil for an earache, a metal coin over an umbilical hernia to reduce the hernia, rice water to maintain electrolyte balance in an infant with diarrhea, teas to relieve abdominal discomfort, warm smoke for the pain associated with earache and colic, ice packs for ankle sprains, mustard plasters for muscle strains, prayer for the removal of hexes, moist herbal packets for broken bones, or coining to release spirits and relieve pain. It is the nurse's responsibility to acknowledge the existence of such practices, to encourage patients' participation in their health care, and to develop with patients treatment plans that incorporate nursing's practice protocols and the patients' belief models. These collaborative nurse-patient plans can help to develop respect and trust between the partners.

An example from my own experience of entering into a collaborative partnership with a mother whose health beliefs were different from my own provides an illustration of how one might combine nursing protocols with a patient's alternative health practices. First, it was important for me to recognize the problem as the mother identified it—her baby had a protruding umbilicus. I recognized the child's condition as a nonthreatening, reducible, nonstrangulating umbilical hernia. Second, I realized that the mother felt that the hernia was unsightly. I felt that the umbilical hernia did not contain abdominal contents, was in no way life threatening, and would more than likely resolve spontaneously once the child began to walk. The mother wanted it to disappear *immediately,* however, and this was the reason she had placed a compress, made with a metal coin inside a thin cloth diaper, over it. In addition, the mother made every effort to keep the baby from crying, because the increased abdominal pressure caused the hernia to protrude even more. On this one issue, the need to prevent the infant from crying excessively, we agreed. For me, the most important things were to keep the infant's skin clean and dry, to prevent erosion of the skin surface under the dressing; to allow for adequate ventilation to the area; and to prevent infection. In order to work cooperatively with the mother, I initially restated her concerns to her in order to make sure I understood her need. Next, I clearly explained to her what my concerns were, and together we agreed upon a plan of care that incorporated my instructions on skin care and her continued use of the abdominal compress. We mutually agreed that she would change the dressing frequently and clean the baby's skin with each diaper change; that she would remove the dressing at the child's bedtime and when the child slept during the day, to accomplish aeration of the area; and that she would take care to see that the dressing did not impede circulation. In addition, I attempted to show the mother, through drawings, the physiological mechanism responsible for the appearance of an umbilical hernia. In conclusion, we established a treatment plan we could both adhere to—my nursing responsibility for the delivery of safe care as well as the mother's need to practice her health beliefs were realized.

Now that I am more autonomous in the management of my clinic time and more flexible in my practice, it has been my experience that the most successful outcomes I have witnessed have always been ones in which patients have taken an active role in the development of their individualized plans of care. Although initially such negotiations added an additional 5 to 10 minutes to office visits, on subsequent visits most patients were more forthcoming with information, the level of trust was elevated, an element of familiarity prevailed, and patients' perceptions of their care were much more positive.

SOCIAL KNOWLEDGE

The phrase "feminization of poverty," introduced by Pearce and McAdoo (1981), aptly makes a connection between women and poverty that is indicative of the social and economic conditions that affect women as a group. Women, as well as children, are the primary beneficiaries of social welfare programs for the poor. In 1980, the poor in the United States were predominantly female. More than half of the families who were poor were headed by women (Ehrenreich & Piven, 1984). The most significant characteristic of female-headed households is their poverty (Moore & Burt, 1982).

On the issues of poverty and health care, one respondent, Sydney, shared this story about the fate of some of the women in her neighborhood: "In this area, a lot of women really won't seek medical help because of their living conditions or their situations in life. When they do go, they're more or less frowned upon. Instead of going though that process, they'd rather have people at home 'doctoring' on the kids." Val wants the best for her child, but can't always get it: "I feel angry and depressed when I can't get what my child needs. It messes with my self-esteem. My growing children are not getting the type of medicine they need and it takes longer for generic medicine to work."

From these comments it is evident that some poor women pay a hefty price for their triple minority status—being poor, female, and ethnic minority. Financial and cultural barriers to service too often negatively influence their lives. In a truly democratic society, the knowledge and practices leading to better health standards and prolonged life in one sector of society must be shared among all citizens (Gordon-Bradshaw, 1987).

As the majority of my patients' incomes fall below the state's definition of poverty (a family of four members with a gross yearly income of less than $20,000 U.S.), it is my practice to advocate for housing, clothing, food, and appropriate medical care for them. On a given day, it is not unusual to learn of at least one homeless family that is in need of safe shelter. In order to meet the needs of these families, my clinic keeps available a list of support organizations, medical referrals, food and clothing closets, and information on inexpensive transportation, and a clinic room is always well stocked with the necessities of life. The entire staff is alert to any news of possible contributions and maintains a constant vigil to locate families who have "slipped through the cracks." As individuals, clinic personnel also make contributions in the forms of money, transportation, food, clothing, child care, elder care, shelter, and emotional support.

I have also come to recognize the value of collaborative practice. On several occasions, as the case manager of a multidisciplinary team consisting of social workers, public health nurses, health aides, and bilingual interpreters, I have conducted individually scheduled provider home visits in order to make more inclusive evaluations of my patients. An example of this practice is a visit I made to the home of Maria, the wife of an unemployed migrant worker. Maria presented at the clinic with two male children: a malnourished, developmentally delayed 6-month-old and an extremely shy, quiet, and slender 3-year-old. During the history intake phase of the visit, through a Spanish interpreter, Maria stated that she was afraid her breast milk was not good enough for her baby. She said she usually ate one meal a day consisting of a tortilla, beans, and a little meat. Her dietary intake had been substantially decreased, not only because money was scarce but also because the family had taken in another migrant family of six people who were unable to contribute financially to the household expenses. In his despair, Maria's husband had started to drink excessively and was becoming increasingly abusive toward her and their 3-year-old son. Neither family had sought government assistance for housing, food, and medical care because they feared their illegal alien status would be revealed, resulting in deportation to Mexico. Maria came to the clinic because she was afraid her 6-month-old child was gravely ill. Had it not been for the inhabitants of the community recognizing the clinic as a safe place and recommending it to her, Maria's situation might have gone unnoticed as she and her family continued to travel from county to county in search of work in the fields.

In order to address this family's basic need for shelter, food, and safety, a multidisciplinary approach to problem solving was put into play to attend to the family's health care needs and to locate work, subsidized housing, clothing, and food. Counseling and parenting assistance were implemented in an attempt to provide a safe, nurturing environment for the children. Maria's husband received counseling related to his abusive behavior and his ineffective coping mechanisms. Maria was instructed on culturally specific mechanisms of empowerment, nutrition, child care, and child growth and development, and on ways to access the health care system.

As a result of this multidisciplinary practice involving the family's participation, Maria's nutritional status improved along with the infant's and older child's growth and development. The family began to thrive and was able to maintain a relatively harmonious existence. At the conclusion of the harvest, the family moved on to pursue work in another area.

CONCLUSION

For poor families, the response to inequity and deprivation is a quest for power, control, and self-ownership. The responses to resistance to inequality are further alienation, rejection, and conflict (Gordon-Bradshaw, 1987). To influence lifestyle and behavior, health promoters must take into account the values, attitudes, culture, and life circumstances of the individual. Therefore, if we are to achieve salutary changes in the health status of all people, health professionals and the designers of health programs must cope with the extraordinary diversity existing in most societies (Nickens, 1990). Moreover, nurses in practice contexts can draw upon the perceptions of their patients and their reflective interpretations of shared experiences to develop useful knowledge and devise new strategies aimed toward a truly emancipatory practice.

REFERENCES

Ehrenreich, B., & Piven, F. F. (1984). The persistence of poverty 1: The feminization of poverty. *Dissent, 31,* 162-170.

Gordon-Bradshaw, R. H. (1987). A social essay on special issues facing poor women of color. *Women & Health, 12,* 243-259.

Griffin, F. N. U. (1994). Perceptions of African American women regarding health care. *Journal of Cultural Diversity, 1*(2), 32-35.

Kupperschmidt, B. (1988). Culturally sensitive nursing care for black clients. *Oklahoma Nurse, 33*(5), 9-18.

LaGuerre, M. (1987). *Afro-Caribbean folk medicine.* South Hadley, MA: Bergin & Garvey.

Moore, K. A., & Burt, M. R. (1982). *Private crisis, public cost: Policy perspectives on teenage childbearing.* Washington, DC: Urban Institute Press.

Nickens, H. W. (1990). Health promotion and disease prevention among minorities. *Health Affairs, 9*(2), 133-143.

Pearce, D., & McAdoo, H. P. (1981). *Women and children, alone and in poverty.* Washington, DC: National Advisory Council on Economic Opportunity.

Rempusheski, V. F. (1989). The role of ethnicity in elder care. *Nursing Clinics of North America, 24,* 717-731.

Tripp-Reimer, R. T., & Larry, A. A. (1989). Cross-cultural perspectives on patient teaching. *Nursing Clinics of North America, 24,* 613-619.

White, J. L., & Parham, T. A. (1990). *The psychology of blacks: An African-American perspective* (2nd ed.). Englewood Cliffs, NJ: Prentice Hall.

Searching for Family Nursing Practice Knowledge

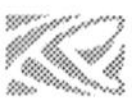

VIRGINIA E. HAYES

I hold a specific perspective about the provision of nursing care, and that is that we, as professional nurses, have a mandate to provide care for families, not just in settings where families are formally recognized (as in pediatric, maternity, and community settings, or as family nurse practitioners in the United States), but also as we care for individuals. Even when a nursing action seems highly focused on individual need (such as changing a dressing, monitoring blood gases, or giving medications), the recipient's family may be directly or indirectly affected by that action. I embrace a concept of family nursing wherein "family" is thought of as context for the individual, wherein the individual is sometimes context for the family, and wherein the family as a whole may be the recipient of care (Friedemann, 1989; Gilliss, 1989; Robinson, 1995; Wright & Leahey, 1990). It is in the family where all of us learn how to be healthy, and when we are not healthy, the family influences and is influenced by our illness, whether it is acute or chronic, sudden or anticipated (Doherty & Campbell, 1988; Ross, Mirowsky, & Goldsteen, 1990). Nurses influence family responses to health and illness through direct and indirect interventions with individuals and aggregates.

Despite the personal convictions of the many nurses who share these views, family nursing practice remains an ill-articulated entity. Why is this? There is a wealth of family theory from several disciplines available to us on which to base our care, a growing conscientiousness about the inclusion of family nursing in undergraduate and graduate curricula, and a burgeoning literature about family considerations in nursing care. However, many of the publications concerned with family nursing have been based on research rather than practice (Bell, 1995a; Ganong, 1995; Hayes, 1993; Whall & Loveland-Cherry, 1993), and, with one or two notable exceptions, consistent use of established family *nursing* theory is not yet evident. There are few sources available to practitioners to guide the integrated processes of caring for families, little concern with family/nurse or nursing/environment/health, and few templates, examples, or overt strategies for thinking about family nursing processes per se.

Despite Western society's and the nursing discipline's apparent valuing of family and the interactions between family and health, knowledge about an entity called "family nursing" has been largely unarticulated. Practicing nurses "know" that family nursing exists in daily practice, albeit in a wide variety of forms, but nurse scholars, educators, researchers, theorists, and practitioners alike have barely begun to grapple with what family nursing is, how it is evidenced, how to study it, how to conceptualize and explain its processes, and even how to do it. I suggest that our disciplinary knowledge has failed so far to capture the interconnected nature of family nursing theory/practice, that is, the knowledge we gain formally through constructs (the preexisting ideas of others) and the experiential knowledge we gain through doing. Further, there are elements of our practical nursing knowledge about which we are theoretically unaware. In my experience, few nurses who consider themselves to be nursing families make evident—to themselves or others—the purposeful, self-conscious thinking that directs the manner in which they act and interact with others as they deliver care. The processing of family nursing knowledge is assumed, taken for granted. Thus in this chapter I examine some of the theory and practice roots of family nursing, with an eye to determining areas for development toward improving the care of families. Although I intend to demonstrate that theoretical and practical family knowledge ought to be considered interactive and inseparable, I will begin by considering them separately, as they are typically addressed within the literature.

FAMILY NURSING THEORY KNOWLEDGE

As members of a practice discipline, nurses cannot act without knowledge or have knowledge without action. These are the reciprocal elements of family nursing practice. To deal with the first part first requires a critical examination of the theoretical bases of family nursing. Currently, this "formal" nursing knowledge (Pryjmachuk, 1996) about families in health care originates from a wide range of sources, primarily in family science and the social sciences. In-the-field experience and current nursing literature testify to the use of a potpourri of theoretical constructs to direct practice. Essentially, whether they are at macro, midrange, or micro levels, these can be classified as either nursing-specific theory or nonnursing theory.

Nonnursing Family Theory

Developing steadily over the past 100 years, family theorizing has reached immense proportions, supported by a dozen or more periodicals and a quantity of book publications every year (Klein & Jurich, 1993). Although the publication list is long, Klein and Jurich (1993) suggest that theoretical achievements are meager. Their assessment is that much family theory is narrowly focused, elitist (in that there is a history in the field of honoring "superstar" theorists), American (despite the fact that family work is also progressing in Europe, South and Central America, Australia, and other parts of the world), positivist, and poorly linked to its location in social and interactional contexts. History has revealed that particular theories become popular without empirical evidence to support their success clinically or in research. At various times in the history of family theorizing, there has been more or less diversity among theories and more or less conflict about their usefulness.

In family nursing, we are influenced by these breezes blowing in the wider family field. Currently, systems, interactionist, ecological, developmental, social exchange, and stress and coping theories are those most frequently cited as the basis for nursing action and research (McShane, 1991; Mercer, 1989), reflecting their popularity in the research and practice of other disciplines. If family nursing continues to follow interdisciplinary trends, we can expect interest in theories as diverse as critical, feminist, conflict, life-course or life-span, social-cognitive-behavioral, communication, and biosocial approaches—frameworks that are more contextually related and capable of addressing ethnicity, race, and oppression. Each of these theoretical constructions has its strengths and weaknesses, and all can be more or less useful in guiding practice, depending on the substantive area of application as well as the philosophical beliefs of the individual practitioner and the practice setting. Our challenge is to become more overtly aware of those principles we embrace in acting and interacting with family members, and to be critically conscious of their influence on health outcomes—from the perspectives of family members themselves (Durand, 1993). As one example, systems theory and its variants are frequently cited as practice frameworks (Sills & Hall, 1985; Stuart, 1991). Complex and intellectually challenging, these theories are seen as intuitively appealing ways to think about families, which are themselves complex and highly varied. Because their language and constructs are cumbersome, however, they invite partial applications that are more heuristic than conceptually cohesive. Despite criticisms leveled against systems theories for their hierarchical structuralist roots (Suppe & Jacox, 1985), mechanistic worldview (Hartrick, 1995), and patriarchal orientation (Whitchurch & Constantine, 1993), they seem to offer nurses an appealing way to think about families and the effects of their care. Indeed, systems thinking is so prevalent in our lives generally that it has become part of our taken-for-granted or "background" knowledge, and only conscientious thinking can tease out the assumptions it creates within us. Only when we become aware of systems thinking can we evaluate its impact.

The same could be said for many other formal frameworks presented in nursing education and literature as ways to think about families and family intervention. All help us conceive some elements of structure, function, growth, development, or interaction within the family unit and between it and the environment. An additional problem is that, as "borrowed" theories, they do not deal directly with concepts elemental to *nursing* practice, such as health, therapeutic relationships, human suffering, and nursing care. None is based on observations of, or reflections on, the experiences of families and nurses with health and illness; that is, the constructs are applied to nursing without formally conceptualized "bridges," and each nurse must make his or her own interpretations to apply them to practice.

Family Nursing Theory

Family nursing theory does little to fill the gaps between concepts and nursing care. Very young in its development (Artinian, 1991; Whall, 1993), family nursing theory progressed slowly in the 1950s, 1960s, and 1970s as early grand theorists focused exclusively on the individual as the recipient of care. Although issues of family care have now become explicit in several existing nursing frameworks (Ross & Cobb, 1990; Whall & Fawcett, 1991), conceptual guidance for interventions with whole families or individuals as members of families and communities remains scarce and problematic (Friedemann, 1989; Gilliss, Roberts, Highley, & Martinson, 1989; Murphy, 1986). This is not to say that family nursing scholars have been silent—quite the contrary—but whereas discussion of isolated issues associated with the care of families is common within the literature, consideration of theoretical patterns having to do with family nursing is rare. For example, although family nursing research is reported, there are few established programs of research in which family nursing concepts are being systematically studied and tied into theory (Ganong, 1995; Hayes, 1993; Whall & Loveland-Cherry, 1993). Very few utilization studies "complete the circle" to practice application. Although opinion articles about the nursing care of families are plentiful, they are rarely linked overtly to theory of any kind and are unsubstantiated by research. Thus there are almost no linkages among published research, theory, and family nursing practice. It is my view that this leaves practicing nurses, even though they may be up-to-date on the literature in their fields, with piecemeal understandings of family nursing and little consistent direction for the focus of their family interventions.

Noteworthy exceptions in the development of family nursing theory are the team of Wright, Leahey, and Bell at the Calgary Family Nursing Unit in Alberta, Canada (Wright, Watson, & Bell, 1990), and Friedemann (1995) at the University of Michigan in the United States. The theoretical outcomes of these scholars' work are based on preexisting established systems theory, clinical practice outcomes systematically observed and documented, and some empirical research. Both Wright et al. and Friedemann consider family members *and* families-as-units to be the recipients of care and aim to work in therapeutic relationships focused on goals that family members assist in setting. In the work of these scholars, theory is thoughtfully considered and practiced, clearly articulated, and viewed as emergent.

In summary, then, much of what family nurses know from formal theory is "borrowed," derived from traditional, positivist assumptions, based on observations with families experiencing difficulties, and aimed at explanation, prediction, and control of events and phenomena (Durand, 1993). Despite great strides in family nursing scholarship, it is rare to find identification of the theory that directs nursing interventions. The nursing of individuals as members of families and of families-as-units is going on—every day, everywhere. I suggest that, in their care of families, nurses take for granted both what they know from theory and what they have learned through experience in practice.

FAMILY NURSING PRACTICE KNOWLEDGE

Whether it is generated outside or inside the discipline, existing theory does not explain all of the ways nurses interact with families in health care. To take up the second part of the statement that we cannot act without knowledge or have knowledge without action, I turn to the nature of knowledge about family nursing that is embedded in how nurses practice with families. How can we talk about this, when it is largely unwritten (Bell, 1995b) and is rarely even spoken (White, 1995)? Fragments of practice knowledge are discernible in teacher-student exchanges in clinical areas, in mentoring exchanges, and in some of the case studies and opinion articles published in the nursing literature. Even when we consider the evidence from such sources, we see that family nurses' practical knowledge is essentially unexplored. As Boyd (1993) points out, "Nursing situations as they are lived through by practicing nurses" are ill understood and certainly under-researched (p. 9).

Johnson (1994) and White (1995) note that practice knowledge, or the "art-acts" of nursing, has received much less systematic attention by nurse scholars tracing nursing's epistemological roots than have other forms of knowing. This less quantifiable knowledge of nursing has been unacknowledged and trivialized until recently (Brykczynski, 1993). I suggest that our inattentiveness to our practical family nursing knowledge contributes to its undervaluing, thus perpetuating a cycle; because it is not valued it is unexplored and unacknowledged, and because it is invisible it is undervalued and minimized.

Because practical family nursing knowledge is relatively unrecognized, unarticulated, and trivialized, we may be unprepared for the outcomes associated with the discovery of practical knowledge. Even though we acknowledge that formal knowing is only part of the picture of the care of family members and families, we tend to be at ease with scientific or theoretical knowledge. However, important elements of good family care are missing from open scrutiny, unexplained by research findings, out-of-discipline theory, and family nursing theory. Discovering the facts, values, and processes of practical family nursing knowledge attributes a value to them, a significant shift from prevalent thinking in the field. The sharing of practical family knowledge among nursing colleagues offers access to ways in which complex decisions about care are made and carried out (Benner, 1994; Benner, Tanner, & Chesla, 1992). The knowledge we discover will undoubtedly be complex and detailed, requiring new ways to organize it and a vocabulary to talk about it. It will require distinct evaluation criteria (Bournaki & Germain, 1993). Nurses will require new skills to construct and reconstruct confidently the output of their reflections about their individual practice (Maeve, 1994).

If we are to recognize, articulate, and value family nursing knowledge, we will need to develop "uncovering methods." To discover family nursing know-how, we must tease out the bases of our family-related care behavior through critical examination of our own beliefs and values, as reflected in our actions, and of others' beliefs and values, as apparent in their actions (Lewis, 1995; Wright, Bell, Watson, & Tapp, 1995). We need to listen to and reflect upon family members' expressed ideas about nursing care (Durand, 1993). Further, we need to process our experiences conscientiously and methodically in providing everyday care for families. This will help to uncover what Johnson (1975) calls commonsense or cultural knowledge, the basis of all knowledge and theory, in his view. Many years of habit, inherited from the positivist tradition, of minimizing the value of commonsense knowledge in favor of "objective" reality must be overcome through innovative methods suitable to making practitioners' subjective reality more visible. To render practice knowledge less obscure, we will need to generate "nonresearch" ways of inquiry. Because concepts related to families, nursing, and the environments in which their interactions take place are highly complex, this will present a significant challenge for family nurses.

Some elements of nursing "art-acts" will probably always be inaccessible to our understanding, whereas other elements may be more accessible than is commonly assumed (White, 1995). Simultaneously, theoretical family knowledge may be both self-evident and obscure. If we accept the premise that these two forms of knowledge are inextricably linked, what techniques might we use to discover the complex bases of family nursing knowledge? Can we uncover significantly more about the how, why, and what-is-it of family nursing practice?

DISCOVERING FAMILY NURSING PRACTICE

I believe that, if we can make such discoveries, more family nursing practice knowledge may be accessible than was previously thought, and family health care will benefit. I propose five means to aid the uncovering of family nursing knowledge: observation, reflection, storytelling, writing and publication, and nontraditional research.

Observation in nursing almost goes without saying—nurses are excellent observers, honing better and better skills of observation as they become more experienced (Benner et al., 1992). To be able to discover some of what lies at the roots of family nursing, nurses must have good observational abilities: abilities to see, pay attention, selectively focus, remember what was seen, and recall it later. To uncover embedded nursing knowledge, nurses must be able to become consciously aware of what is being thought and done, by themselves and by others.

The value of conscientious, thoughtful *reflection* in uncovering the art of nursing has been the subject of an increasing number of recent publications (Greenwood, 1995; Powell, 1989; Richardson, 1993). Reflection is simply thinking—an everyday, mundane occurrence. In the context of discovering nursing practice knowledge, however, it takes on the connotation of purposefulness, of "the turning back of the experience of the individual upon himself" (Mead, as quoted in Greenwood, 1995, p. 1045). To discover practice-based knowledge of family nursing actions or to locate taken-for-granted theoretical concepts, reflection must be conscious and conscientious. Schön (1983) terms this "reflection-in-action" and "reflection-on-action," that is, thinking carefully about family interventions both while we are doing them and after we have done them. Once a nurse's consciousness is raised about the interactive processes of observing and reflecting about her or his actions, she or he will become increasingly reflective while delivering care as well as in quiet moments afterward (while traveling home after work, exercising, and so on). For example, I might become puzzled about, interested in, or aware of why I organized the baths of toddlers in a four-bed ward in the order I did, given the existing combination of factors: intravenous drips, vital signs, feedings, medications to give, and the presence of two mothers, one obviously cranky and sleepy, and one quiet with staff but interactive with her son. I would ask myself a series of questions about my actions and others' responses to them, and reflect on the ideas that these uncover. Schön notes that the twin abilities of reflection-in-action and reflection-on-action can be improved through training and feedback, such as with a skilled teacher or mentor, but that increased awareness and practice/experience may serve as well.

Unlike Maeve (1994), I see *storytelling* and reflection as somewhat different, though their "chicken or the egg" nature could be debated. They may form a continuous loop, wherein a nurse selects a story representative of family nursing upon reflection and then, in telling the story, reflects upon its elements and reconstructs its meaning. The clinical stories of nursing practice with families are like Benner et al.'s (1992) exemplars, and tend to be complex and multilayered. Family care explanations, assertions, and descriptions are likely to be multiple, varied in degree of complexity, and a mixture of theoretical and commonsense knowledge. Chinn (1989) notes that it is important that both stories and the reflection on them (or on story components) emphasize "lived experience and the significance of everyday life" (p. 74), that is, the everyday life of both the nurse and the family or family member, as well as any other people who are involved.

Writing turns entirely mental representations into semantic, concrete representations that are accessible to others or to ourselves again at another time. When we capture our insights about family practice in story or reflective form and write them down, we discover the experiential and theoretical knowledge from which nursing actions spring. Journals and diaries are personal and private ways in which to capture such discoveries. Newsletters, conference workshops and presentations, and *publication* in periodicals are among a range of more formal and public ways to share reflected clinical knowledge with others.

Nontraditional research is the final strategy I recommend for discovering family nursing practice knowledge. The usual means of "doing science" have not captured and will not capture the knowledge of practice, whatever its bases (Boyd, 1993; Pryjmachuk, 1996). The almost intangible, barely verbal, highly abstract, and complex knowledge that produces family interventions requires innovative, "out of the box" approaches to documenting, recording, analyzing, and summarizing. Interpretive, participatory, and feminist methods spring to mind, but the study of the nature and sources of practice knowledge will demand methods that have not yet been conceived. I see these as varying from self-investigatory practices (such as heuristic research) that could be used by individual nurses to group methods that could combine "data" from individuals and collectives. They will need to encompass ways to question both systematically and creatively, to record, and to examine family knowledge from nurses representing all levels of expertise in order to identify some of the theory embedded in practice and the practice knowledge embedded in practice—a challenge for future family nurse scholars.

These five strategies for uncovering some of the theory/practice of family nursing are not exhaustive; I offer them to begin a dialogue about ways to pursue the roots of family nursing knowledge. The products of conscientious exploration for the explanations of family nursing will, in my opinion, include the following: increased awareness of the how-tos and the whys of care actions; valuing of experiential or art-act knowledge about families in health care; increased clarity about the objectives of care; increased effectiveness of interventions and, possibly more important, increased ability to evaluate their effectiveness; increased confidence and satisfaction with care; and more authoritative functioning in all aspects of the multidisciplinary team, including program and policy planning. An accessible body of family nursing practice knowledge will therefore result in an improvement of the quality and quantity of family nursing care.

DEVELOPING A CRITICAL CONSCIOUSNESS

Although there is now a significant body of literature in the area of family nursing, and research reports reveal an impressive engagement with nursing-related family issues, it is unclear how this body of formal knowledge directs nursing interventions. Meanwhile, experiential or practical family nursing knowledge is essentially obscure from ourselves, our colleagues, and the recipients of our care. This chapter is a call to those to those who value our contributions to the nursing of families to analyze critically the roots of how and why we do the things we do in our care for whole families and for the members of families. The scope of this self-analysis and criticism must extend beyond the traditional spheres of research and theory development called for by Gilliss and Davis (1992) to include as well the discovery of practice knowledge embedded within the everyday actions of nurses and families in health care. To modify an image from Doherty, Boss, LaRossa, Schumm, and Steinmetz (1993), from their introduction to their multidisciplinary sourcebook of developing theories and methods for the study of families:

> The contemporary challenge in [understanding family nursing], then, is to become more critically reflective in order to discern what we are saying about ourselves and what we are saying about the families. . . . It is as though we look through a two-way mirror at families. When the light is turned on the families, we see them through the medium of the glass. When the lights are switched to our side, we see ourselves and our surroundings reflected in the mirror—and we become visible to the families and their communities. In future we must become more adept at switching the lights back and forth. (p. 27)

While the lights are on on our side of the glass, we need to look to see what we see of ourselves, because gaining self-awareness will in turn help us focus on families so as to provide care that is meaningful and effective for them.

Because most health care goes on within the family, families are extremely valuable to society and to health care delivery systems worldwide. It is in the family that individuals learn to be healthy and to cope with situations that deviate from health. Nurses touch families' responses to health and illness only during the time when individuals or families-as-units formally enter the delivery system. It is our entrusted responsibility to make the most of those periods of "touch." To take this seriously, we need to examine the roots of our practice consciously and conscientiously, what is formally known and informally known as well as what can be made visible through how we act with families and family members. The "critical consciousness" stance that I advocate reflects the valuing of both families and nursing through examination of the assumptions and explanations about care that we tend to take for granted. The strategies I have suggested here for capturing the interrelated ways we know and nurse families are just a beginning. Recapturing old and discovering new ways to uncover the bases of our care will lead to increasingly sophisticated and applicable insights about families in health care and will result in improved family nursing. This influence on families and their members' health is an important nursing contribution to society: action with a purpose.

REFERENCES

Artinian, N. T. (1991). Philosophy of science and family nursing theory development. In A. L. Whall & J. Fawcett (Eds.), *Family theory development in nursing: State of the science and art* (pp. 43-54). Philadelphia: Davis.

Bell, J. M. (1995a). Family nursing network: A place to communicate and exchange ideas about family nursing: It's a small world. *Journal of Family Nursing, 1,* 352.

Bell, J. M. (1995b). Wanted: family nursing interventions. *Journal of Family Nursing, 1,* 355-358.

Benner, P. (1994). Response to "Practice theories in nursing and science of nursing practice." *Scholarly Inquiry for Nursing Practice, 8,* 159-162.

Benner, P., Tanner, C., & Chesla, C. (1992). From beginner to expert: Gaining a differentiated clinical world in critical care nursing. *Advances in Nursing Science, 14,* 13-28.

Bournaki, M.-C., & Germain, C. P. (1993). Esthetic knowledge in family-centered nursing care of hospitalized children. *Advances in Nursing Science, 16*(2), 81-89.

Boyd, C. A. (1993). Toward a nursing practice research method. *Advances in Nursing Science, 16*(2), 9-25.

Brykczynski, K. A. (1993). Nurse practitioner-patient discourse: Uncovering the voice of nursing in primary care practice. *Scholarly Inquiry for Nursing Practice, 7,* 159-163.

Chinn, P. L. (1989). Nursing patterns of knowledge and feminist thought. *Nursing and Health Care, 10,* 71-75.

Doherty, W. J., Boss, P. G., LaRossa, R., Schumm, W. R., & Steinmetz, S. K. (1993). Family theories and methods: A contextual approach. In P. G. Boss, W. J. Doherty, R. LaRossa, W. R. Schumm, & S. K. Steinmetz (Eds.), *Sourcebook of family theories and methods: A contextual approach* (pp. 3-30). New York: Plenum.

Doherty, W. J., & Campbell, T. L. (1988). *Families and health.* Newbury Park, CA: Sage.

Durand, B. A. (1993). Preface. In S. L. Feetham, S. B. Meister, J. M. Bell, & C. L. Gilliss (Eds.), *The nursing of families: Theory/research/education/practice* (pp. ix-xiii). Newbury Park, CA: Sage.

Friedemann, M.-L. (1989). The concept of family nursing. *Journal of Advanced Nursing, 14,* 211-214.

Friedemann, M.-L. (1995). *The framework of systemic organization: A conceptual approach to families and nursing.* Thousand Oaks, CA: Sage.

Ganong, L. H. (1995). Current trends and issues in family nursing research. *Journal of Family Nursing, 1,* 171-206.

Gilliss, C. L. (1989). Why family health care? In C. L. Gilliss, B. L. Highley, B. M. Roberts, & I. M. Martinson (Eds.), *Toward a science of family nursing* (pp. 3-8). Menlo Park, CA: Addison-Wesley.

Gilliss, C. L., & Davis, L. L. (1992). Family nursing research: Percepts from paragons and peccadilloes. *Journal of Advanced Nursing, 17,* 28-33.

Gilliss, C. L., Roberts, B. M., Highley, B. L., & Martinson, I. M. (1989). What is family nursing? In C. L. Gilliss, B. L. Highley, B. M. Roberts, & I. M. Martinson (Eds.), *Toward a science of family nursing* (pp. 64-73). Menlo Park, CA: Addison-Wesley.

Greenwood, R. (1995). Humpty Dumpty: Reflection and reflective nursing practice. *Journal of Advanced Nursing, 21,* 1044-1050.

Hartrick, G. A. (1995). Part 1: Transforming family nursing theory: From mechanicism to contextualism. *Journal of Family Nursing, 1,* 134-147.

Hayes, V. E. (1993). Nursing science in family care, 1984-1990. In S. L. Feetham, S. B. Meister, J. M. Bell, & C. L. Gilliss (Eds.), *Advances in the nursing of families* (pp. 18-29). Newbury Park, CA: Sage.

Johnson, J. L. (1994). A dialectical examination of nursing art. *Advances in Nursing Science, 17*(1), 1-14.

Johnson, J. M. (1975). *Doing field research.* New York: Free Press.

Klein, D. M., & Jurich, J. A. (1993). Metatheory and family studies. In P. G. Boss, W. J. Doherty, R. LaRossa, W. R. Schumm, & S. K. Steinmetz (Eds.), *Sourcebook of family theories and methods: A contextual approach* (pp. 31-67). New York: Plenum.

Lewis, E. A. (1995). Toward a tapestry of impassioned voices: Incorporating praxis into teaching about families. *Family Relations, 44,* 149-152.

Maeve, M. K. (1994). The carrier bag theory of nursing practice. *Advances in Nursing Science, 16*(4), 9-22.

McShane, R. E. (1991). Family theoretical perspectives and implications for nursing practice. *AACN Clinical Issues in Critical Care Nursing, 2,* 210-219.

Mercer, R. T. (1989). Theoretical perspectives on the family. In C. L. Gilliss, B. L. Highley, B. M. Roberts, & I. M. Martinson (Eds.), *Toward a science of family nursing* (pp. 9-36). Menlo Park, CA: Addison-Wesley.

Murphy, S. (1986). Family study and nursing research. *Image: The Journal of Nursing Scholarship, 18,* 170-174.

Powell, J. H. (1989). The reflective practitioner in nursing. *Journal of Advanced Nursing, 14,* 824-832.

Pryjmachuk, S. (1996). A nursing perspective on the interrelationships between theory, research and practice. *Journal of Advanced Nursing, 23,* 679-684.

Richardson, J. (1993). Reflective practice: A critique of the work of Argyris and Schön. *Journal of Advanced Nursing, 18,* 1183-1187.

Robinson, C. A. (1995). Beyond dichotomies in the nursing of persons and families. *Image: The Journal of Nursing Scholarship, 27,* 116-120.

Ross, B., & Cobb, K. L. (1990). *Family nursing: A nursing process approach.* Redwood City, CA: Addison-Wesley.

Ross, C. E., Mirowsky, J., & Goldsteen, K. (1990). The impact of the family on health: The decade in review. *Journal of Marriage and the Family, 52,* 1059-1078.

Schön, D. A. (1983). *The reflective practitioner.* New York: Basic Books.

Sills, G. M., & Hall, J. E. (1985). A general systems perspective for nursing. In J. E. Hall & B. R. Weaver (Eds.), *Distributive nursing practice: A systems approach to community health* (pp. 21-29). Philadelphia: J. B. Lippincott.

Stuart, M. E. (1991). An analysis of the concept of family. In A. L. Whall & J. Fawcett (Eds.), *Family theory development in nursing: State of the science and art* (pp. 31-42). Philadelphia: Davis.

Suppe, F., & Jacox, A. K. (1985). Philosophy of science and the development of nursing theory. *Annual Review of Nursing Research, 3,* 241-267.

Whall, A. L. (1993). Disciplinary issues related to family theory development in nursing. In S. L. Feetham, S. B. Meister, J. M. Bell, & C. L. Gilliss (Eds.), *The nursing of families: Theory/research/education/practice* (pp. 13-17). Newbury Park, CA: Sage.

Whall, A. L., & Fawcett, J. (1991). The family as a focal phenomenon in nursing. In A. L. Whall & J. Fawcett (Eds.), *Family theory development in nursing: State of the science and art* (pp. 7-29). Philadelphia: Davis.

Whall, A. L., & Loveland-Cherry, C. J. (1993). Family unit-focused research: 1984-1991. In J. J. Fitzpatrick, R. L. Taunton, & A. S. Jacox (Eds.), *Annual review of nursing research* (pp. 227-247). New York: Springer.

Whitchurch, G. G., & Constantine, L. L. (1993). Systems theory. In P. G. Boss, W. J. Doherty, R. LaRossa, W. R. Schumm, & S. K. Steinmetz (Eds.), *Sourcebook of family theory and methods* (pp. 325-352). New York: Plenum.

White, J. (1995). Patterns of knowing: Review, critique, and update. *Advances in Nursing Science, 17*(1), 73-86.

Wright, L. M., Bell, J. M., Watson, W. L., & Tapp, D. M. (1995). The influence of the beliefs of nurses: A clinical example of a post-myocardial-infarction couple. *Journal of Family Nursing, 1,* 238-256.

Wright, L. M., & Leahey, M. (1990). Trends in nursing families. *Journal of Advanced Nursing, 15,* 148-154.

Wright, L. M., Watson, W. L., & Bell, J. M. (1990). The family nursing unit: A unique integration of research, education, and clinical practice. In J. M. Bell, W. L. Watson, & L. M. Wright (Eds.), *The cutting edge of family nursing* (pp. 95-112). Calgary, AB: Family Nursing Unit Publications.

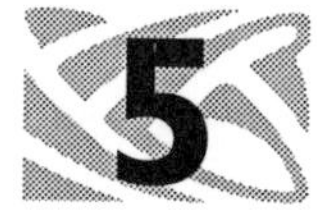

Knowing and Forgetting

The Challenge of Technology for a Reflexive Practice Science of Nursing

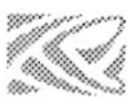

MARGARETE SANDELOWSKI

Scholars of nursing became particularly intrigued with exploring "patterns of knowing" other than science after Carper's (1978) now-classic paper appeared on the subject (e.g., Chinn, 1989; Chinn & Watson, 1994; Jacobs-Kramer & Chinn, 1988; White, 1995; Wolfer, 1993). However, technology, as a way of knowing in nursing, has yet to draw much scholarly attention. Although conventionally seen in its immediate and obvious mode of manifestation as physical object (Mitcham, 1994, pp. 160-161), technology is also a way in which human beings come to know reality, nature, or the world. The word *technology* etymologically contains thought (*logos*) and connotes knowledge (Layton, 1974). Technology is "a practical engagement with the world" (Rothenberg, 1993, p. xvi) accomplished through the making ("bringing into existence") and using ("putting into practice") of artifacts (Mitcham, 1994, p. 231). As a kind of praxis, or thoughtful action, technology is knowing of, in, and through doing.

Although technology has long contributed to nursing praxis, the serious consideration of technology *as knowledge* is still largely restricted to the field of nursing informatics and to discussions concerning knowledge about and of, as opposed to knowledge in and through, technology. The relative lack of philosophical or historical consideration of the intellectual component of technology in nursing is significant because it is implicated in the invisibility of nursing practice *as praxis* and in the denial of and even flight from the "merely" manual or technical in nursing (Dickoff & James, 1992a, p. 573). There remains a pervasive, culturally derived tendency in and out of nursing to ignore, trivialize, and even denigrate procedures involving the hands and devices as nothing more than medically dependent and robotic techniques that can be performed by virtually anyone. There is also a tendency to devalue the know-how involved in executing these procedures (Dickoff & James, 1992a, 1992b; Layton, 1974).

Although there have been important recent efforts to recover and revalorize the everyday, concrete, material, and flesh-and-blood world of nursing practice (e. g., Benner, 1984; Wolf, 1986), there remains a reluctance to define the essence of nursing as located in the body (Cheek & Rudge, 1994, p. 21) and in the physical world. Eager to escape any form of subservience, and particularly the kind of subservience associated with "applied" knowledge and the visceral nature of everyday nursing practice, scholars of nursing have sought to locate the essence of nursing in the "purity" and "nobility" of mental abstractions, or "basic" scientific knowledge (Dickoff & James, 1992a, 1992b).

In this chapter, I consider technology as a distinctive way of knowing in nursing that is fundamental to nursing practice and fundamentally related to empirical, ethical, aesthetic, and personal patterns of knowing. I also consider the challenges that the epistemic relations (Ihde, 1979) between human beings and machines pose for nursing practice. Although technology has modes of manifestation other than as "knowledge" that are not separable from each other—that is, modes of manifestation as "object," "activity," and "volition" (Mitcham, 1994)—I place analytic emphasis here on technology as knowledge.

THE PRIMACY OF TECHNOLOGY

The prevailing idea that technology is merely applied science, or that it constitutes no knowledge itself, has become increasingly less favored among philosophers and social scientists who have found the definition of technology, and the boundaries and relationships between technology and science, to have changed over time (Mitcham, 1994; Wajcman, 1991). Ferguson (1977) observes that the modern assumption that whatever knowledge resides in technology must be derived from science is "a bit of modern folklore" that ignores "non-scientific modes of thought." The many artifacts around us "are as they are" because their makers have established their shapes, styles, and textures. These properties are thought about and visualized in the "mind's eye," but cannot be reduced to verbal description. As Ferguson notes, "Pyramids, cathedrals, and rockets exist not because of geometry, theory of structures, or thermodynamics, but because they were first a picture—literally a vision—in the minds of those who built them" (p. 827).

Ferguson's concern over the denigration of the nonliterary and nonscientific intellectual component of technology calls to mind the recent and varied efforts of nursing scholars to revalorize the often tacit, incommunicable, and aesthetic knowing in nursing. In their efforts to make nursing practice recognized as an important "empirical encounter," Dickoff and James (1992b) similarly lament the lack of recognition of the nonverbal thought involved in doing and of doing itself as a "privileged occasion for expanding knowledge" (p. 580). This failure may partly explain the new attention to the "lost art" (Chinn & Watson, 1994, p. xiv) in and of nursing, where *art* has referred paradoxically both to the technical and the procedural (as in nursing arts) and to what is artful *as opposed to* technical (Chinn & Watson, 1994; Johnson, 1994).

A significant component of doing in nursing has always involved the use of technological objects, a fact of nursing practice that has historically engendered ambivalence and controversy concerning the essence of nursing (for example, as art, practical art, science, or applied science). The incorporation of technology into practice has also engendered debate over whether technology has enhanced or retarded the social and political advancement of nursing. The medical transfer of technology to nursing is variously perceived as having empowered and disempowered nursing (e.g., Fairman, 1992; Melosh, 1982; Sandelowski, 1988; Wagner, 1980; Weeks, 1988).

The (Re)making of Science and Nature

The close tie that now exists between Western technology and science is a fairly recent one, given that what is currently referred to as technology used to be more closely linked to art and craft by virtue of an emphasis on design, aesthetic vision, and skilled making (Ingold, 1988). The idea of the dependency of technology on science became entrenched only after the seventeenth-century revolution in Western science. Emphasizing the actual practice of science, as opposed to its theoretical products, historians and philosophers of science and technology have increasingly challenged the text(story)book image of the relationships among nature, science, and technology. Here, nature poses questions for and is subsequently explained by and mirrored (Rorty, 1979) in science, which, in turn, provides the basis for the technology that is used further to reveal and to control nature (Faulkner, 1994; Ihde, 1991; Rothenberg, 1993). This image can be formalized as follows:

Nature → Science → Technology → Nature

Yet a view of science and technology that may be more in line with historical reality and that emphasizes perception and the concrete practice of science is what Ihde (1991) calls "instrumental realism," a view that gives primacy to technology and one that emphasizes the transformation of nature (or reality or the world) engendered by the technology employed to "reveal" it. This view can be formalized as follows:

Nature_1 → Technology → Science → Nature_2

According to Ihde, modern science is necessarily embodied in technology. The scientific reality intended to correspond to nature is, in actuality, a reality mediated by instruments, such as the telescope and the microscope. An instrumental realist view of modern science emphasizes science as a product of the technology that reveals what science ultimately constructs as reality or nature. As Ihde (1991) argues, it is not technology that is the product or embodiment of science, but rather modern science that is the product of technology and that is "technologically embodied. . . . Instruments form the conditions for and are the mediators of much, if not all, current scientific knowledge" (p. 45). Technological objects permit scientists to see and shape (that is, magnify or reduce) what they see. Science is largely visual (Lynch & Woolgar, 1988) by virtue of the instrumentation that enhances vision and the visual products of this instrumentation (such as photographs, rhythm strips, and graphs).

Moreover, rather than being mirrored in science, nature is itself the product of a technology-dependent science. Nature is as much made as found. Technology is a practical engagement with nature (Nature1) that produces a new nature (Nature2). Rothenberg (1993) observes that the windmill reveals the power of the wind and the shovel discloses the nature of the soil. We grasp the significance of Niagara Falls (nature) because of the tunnel (technology) that brings us closer to it. Yet the Falls, and our relationship with the Falls, are changed by virtue of the tunnel. Technology extends us into the world and, in the process, re-creates it. Technology is thus both revealing and transforming of nature. The nature/technology dichotomy is an outmoded and even false opposition (Channell, 1991). Nature is not so easily separated from artifice as instrument-mediated reality *is nature in a new guise.* Indeed, "what is natural is man's artifice" (Fletcher, 1988, p. 44).

A recurring paradox is that we use technology to reach nature, but always lose it as it was because the very act of reaching for it changes it. Nature is thus always out of human reach, because it is no longer what it was prior to our reaching it. Not only is the nature that we—as part of nature and creators of artifice—strive toward changed by the tools we use, but also our desires and intentions to act in the world, as well as our very experiences of self. Technology extends human capacities and will and, by virtue of that extension, alters them. We (re)invent technology, but technology also reinvents us.

Not only can technology be viewed as having primacy over science, it can also be viewed as independent of science. Contemporary science and technology are intertwined, but many important technological innovations in the past have preceded or owe nothing to science (e.g., White, 1962). Although science is never independent of technology, technology can be independent of science and may have a distinctive epistemology characterized by a practical-artifactual orientation, the central activity of which is design (Faulkner, 1994; Harding, 1991). The relation between technology and art and craft is most visible in design.

TECHNOLOGY AND OTHER WAYS OF KNOWING

Technology is fundamentally related to other ways of knowing or "realms of meaning" (Phenix, 1964). Technology involves the creative and expressive dimensions (Jacobs-Kramer & Chinn, 1988) of empirical, ethical, aesthetic, and personal knowledge. For example, Faulkner (1994, p. 447) has developed a composite typology of knowledge used in technological innovation, including knowledge related to (a) the natural world (such as scientific and engineering theory and the properties of materials); (b) design practice (such as design criteria, concepts, competence, and instrumentalities, and practical experience; (c) research and development; (d) final product (such as operating performance and production competence); and (e) equipment, materials, facilities, and services. In the nursing literature across clinical specialty areas, nurses have variously emphasized knowledge in the practical realm of scientific and technical principles, device operations and maintenance, skilled application of devices to patients, accurate interpretation of device outputs, and artful and ethical integration of devices into practice.

In the Empirical Realm

In the empirical realm, technology is an extension of the sensory or interpretive capacities of its human users; it permits users to create scientific knowledge. A case in point is the technology of prenatal surveillance and diagnosis, which has advanced understanding of fetal development largely by making it more accessible to human sight.

Arguably, the "fetus" as we know it today is what Ihde (1991) refers to in another context as a "technologically carpentered" entity. Similarly, Duden (1993) concludes that the human fetus is no longer the "creature of God or natural fact" it had been for most of human history, but rather an "engineered construct of modern society" (p. 4). The "synthesis" of this new fetus was accomplished largely through prenatal technology. Only recently have women carried fetuses they could "see" (p. 6); only recently has the pregnant woman's "carnal knowledge" (p. 8) of the fetus been supplanted in value by the defleshed knowledge obtained through technology. According to Duden, the story of the "technogenesis of the fetal image" is largely the "history of its visualization" (p. 92). Historically, conceptually, and experientially far removed from the unseen unborn, the fetus is now a technologically constructed entity that can be examined, sampled, and treated as a patient in its own right (Mattingly, 1992).

In the Ethical Realm

Technology is a way of knowing that is fundamentally related to the ethical realm. Whereas technologies are epistemically nonneutral because they transform reality (Ihde, 1979, 1990), they are ethically nonneutral because they reinforce or create moral values, norms, or positions. Technologies have a material and moral side, as they always involve choices concerning the purposes to which they will be put, the desires they will satisfy, the interests they will serve, and their status as means and ends (Bush, 1983; Jonas, 1979; Mitcham, 1994).

For example, intrinsic to the technology of prenatal diagnosis is the capability to see and manipulate the fetus, a feature that reinforces, creates, or affirms the value and rightness of seeking access to and control of the fetus. Physicians have typically lauded their new ability to gain access to the fetus (e.g., Daffos, 1989), but some expectant parents have found this ability morally problematic and have voiced concern over the morality of looking at the fetus in the sanctum of the womb as well as what it is right to look for (Sandelowski & Black, 1994).

In the Aesthetic Realm

Technology is a way of knowing that is fundamentally related to the aesthetic realm by virtue of its design features and aesthetic values. Whether contributing to the design of a device or to the artful integration of devices into practice, nurses' interaction with technology constitutes an important component of the art of nursing: a way to express or embody nursing knowledge and values (Katims, 1993).

Technology gives work and human relations a certain look, sound, and feel—as, for instance, in the machine-age aesthetic of the intensive care unit. Technological objects and environments are often perceived as providing a kind of "aesthetic delight" or discomfort. Indeed, technological objects are examples of how things designed for other than aesthetic purposes can have even greater influence on the "aesthetic consciousness" than what are typically considered works of art (Phenix, 1964, p. 144). In U.S. culture, the car and the gun are important sources of aesthetic experience. Similarly, clinical devices, such as the ultrasound machine, are important sources of aesthetic experience for patients and caregivers, variously stimulating the senses and emotions (e.g., Sandelowski, 1994a, 1994b).

In the Personal Realm

Technology is fundamentally related to personal knowledge (Phenix, 1964). The making and using of technology often involve a comprehension of the whole that may be incommunicable through language. As the primary machine tenders in health care, nurses often acquire an understanding of how to apply, operate, and interpret the products of devices that becomes an integral part of the tacit know-how of clinical practice.

Although human interactions with machines are commonly viewed and experienced as "I-It" relations, they may also involve "I-Thou" relations (Buber, 1958). Personal knowledge can be obtained from "I-Thou" relations with nonperson entities, such as nature or machines. In contrast to "I-It" human-machine relations characterized by objectification, manipulation, and coercion, "I-Thou" relations are characterized by respect and freedom. Technology is often experienced as emancipating and as an enhancement of humanity. Individual machines have been described in animate terms, as "vital" (Channell, 1991), as "fecund" (Tisdale, 1986), as having "a life of their own" (Cowan, 1983), and as having "biographies" (Wiener, Strauss, Fagerhaugh, & Suczek, 1979). Technological objects have also been described as having a "latent language" (Rothenberg, 1993), "latent telic inclinations," and "implicit rhythms" of their own (Ihde, 1979) that can redirect human behavior.

Personal knowledge also includes relations with oneself that may be altered by technology. Devices are often literally, as in the case of joint replacements, or figuratively, as in treating a device as an extension of a person (Starkman, 1976), incorporated into an embodied self, thereby creating new self-understandings. A common self-understanding attributed to medical technology involves persons who think of themselves or others as or like machines. The medicalization of human life and death is typically described in terms of the mechanization or technologizing of human functions and processes (e.g., Davis-Floyd, 1992). When machine monitoring began to enter nursing practice, nurses began to refer to themselves as the real and best monitors (e.g., Minckley, 1968).

The Intertwining of Realms of Meaning

In actual practice, the realms of empirics, ethics, aesthetics, and personal knowledge are intertwined in technology, and in frequently problematic ways. In the case of prenatal diagnosis, a primary value is placed on seeing for the empirical goals of scientific description, explanation, and intervention. Yet the question remains whether prenatal diagnosis objectifies the pregnant woman and the fetus, and whether it satisfies a need to see (for the welfare of the fetus) or merely the desire to see (out of curiosity, or to acquire the power of looking, or for the pleasure of seeing what used to be unseen). Feminist scholarship concerning prenatal technology (e.g., Petchesky, 1987) and cultural studies concerning the dilemmas of display (Stafford,

1993) have suggested the fine line, and even moral fault line, that can exist between scientific observation and pure voyeurism. When nurses employ or deploy technologies such as fetal ultrasonography, they not only traverse several realms of meaning, but are also implicated in the dilemmas raised on this epistemic journey.

THE EPISTEMIC SITUATION OF HUMAN-MACHINE RELATIONS

Ihde's (1979, 1983, 1990, 1991) phenomenology of human-machine relations offers a framework for understanding the distinctive "epistemic situation" of different technologies and how they may differently (in)form nursing practice. Ihde differentiates between in-the-flesh relations, or knowledge of the world obtainable without the use of any artifacts or instruments, and instrument-mediated relations. He formalizes in-the-flesh relations as Human → World. He then describes four kinds of instrument-mediated relations in which knowledge is through, with, of, or within or among technological objects: embodiment relations, hermeneutic relations, alterity relations, and background relations.

Embodiment Relations

In embodiment relations, a device withdraws from or becomes almost transparent to the human experiencer, whose *I* is extended beyond body limits. Ihde formalizes this relation as (Human-technology) → World. Ihde (1979) uses the example of the dental probe, a device that extends the user's tactile intentionality. When a device such as the dental probe functions well, it is hardly noticed by its human user, who experiences it as quasi-me. Yet at the same time that the probe amplifies knowledge by making available information about the tooth that is not available to the naked finger, it reduces knowledge of the tooth only to what can be obtained through the probe. That is, although the probe provides information about the tooth that the unaided finger cannot provide, only the finger can obtain information about the tooth concerning its temperature or moisture.

According to Ihde, it is a principle of human-machine relations that with every amplification of experience made possible by an instrument, there is a simultaneous reduction of experience. For example, an instrument-mediated enhancement of visual access to the fetus via ultrasonography is simultaneously a reduction of knowledge of the fetus to vision: to only what can be seen. We tend to notice technological amplifications or enhancements because they are often perceived as dramatic (hence our awe concerning technology), but we tend to overlook what we have lost as a consequence of these enhancements.

We also become deskilled in the in-the-flesh or simpler instrumental means of knowledge acquisition replaced by more complex instrumentation. In a study I am now conducting concerning technology in nursing, several nurses have noted the gradual loss of the skills of fetal auscultation and uterine palpation, techniques that have been largely replaced by electronic fetal monitoring. (One nurse noted that nurses now have to relearn and use these skills to validate machine-generated information about the fetal heart and maternal contractions.)

In addition, we are tempted to treat instrument-mediated knowledge as more real than in-the-flesh knowledge, especially when that knowledge produces what we take to be documentary evidence of its existence—for example, the ultrasound picture or the rhythm strip. According to Ihde, physical reality in modern science is largely instrument mediated; it is not the reality available to the flesh, or to the finger or eye or other naked sense medium. We have become increasingly unaware of how much our understanding of the world is derived from and irretrievably transformed by this instrumental mediation.

Hermeneutic Relations

In hermeneutic relations, not only is reality transformed by what instruments permit us to know, but the knowledge produced is itself an altered representation of reality. Ihde formalizes this relation as Human → (technology-World). Whereas embodiment relations with machines extend sensory capability, hermeneutic relations extend interpretive capacity.

When nurses appraise patient temperature with a device, they are not engaging in an embodied activity of actually sensing hot or cold (as when they touch a patient's brow), but rather in a hermeneutic activity involving the reading of a text. Nurses learn to read, or interpret, the height of a column of mercury on a glass thermometer or the digital display on an automated temperature device, both of which stand for (but are not directly experienced as) differences in temperature. Hermeneutic relations with machines imply a relationship with devices even more removed from the flesh than embodied relations. That is, knowledge is not obtained from the senses, but rather from interpretive readings of the texts machines produce, such as rhythm strips, numbers, and other visual displays. Such readings require the nurse to separate what is actually real about the patient's condition from what is artifactually real. Machines may misrepresent patient conditions, as when an instrument halves or doubles fetal heart rates.

Alterity Relations

In alterity relations, the otherness or obviousness of a technology is so profound as to be experienced as quasi-other. Ihde formalizes these relations as Human → technology-(-World). There is a stronger sense in alterity relations of interacting with something other than, but having some similarity to, oneself. This quasi-otherness may manifest itself as a kind of quasi-animation or quasi-autonomy, where users positively or negatively experience a device as having a life and will of its own. Ihde (1990) refers to the computer as a strong example of the love-hate relationships often evident in alterity relations with devices and the tendency to animate and even romantically anthropomorphize devices.

As depicted in many fictional treatments of human-machine relations, the machine can be experienced either as a friendly and helpful automaton or as a Frankenstein-like monster gone wild. Beginning in the 1960s, when high technology began to be incorporated seriously into nursing practice, nurses increasingly referred to technology as either master of or slave to the nurse, and voiced concerns that they might be replaced by machines (e.g., Abbey, 1978; "Machines in Perspective," 1965). Nurses continue to voice their concern that the "essence of nursing [not] be robotized" (Brown, 1985, p. iv). (A drawing in an *American Journal of Nursing* article depicted a robot wearing a nursing cap; Bean, Krahn, Anderson, & Yoshida, 1963, p. 66.)

Background Relations

In background human-machine relations, technology is present in its pervasiveness, but absent in its relative invisibility to human beings. The human environment has become increasingly technological, with behind-the-scenes technology such as electrical power, air heating and cooling, and running water in the home and workplace now virtually unnoticed (unless breakdowns occur). In background relations, devices constitute the physical environment human beings inhabit. Indeed, technological environments have become the "natural" habitats of most Westerners and of much caregiving in the home and hospital.

THE EPISTEMIC CHALLENGE OF TECHNOLOGY FOR NURSING

Knowledge is antecedent to, a consequence of, and inherent in technology. Inventors, engineers, and designers must have the knowledge of making, and users must have the knowledge of using. Devices, in interaction with human users, create new, instrument-mediated knowledge and are themselves material manifestations of knowledge. Technology transcends and belies the outmoded polarities that place technology in false opposition to or even in conflict with human nature—that reify distinctions between means and ends, product and process, embodied and disembodied, art and science, and, most notably, thought and action.

The challenge of technology for a reflexive practice science of nursing lies in our recognizing, apprehending the implications of, and then acting on the knowledge transformations technology engenders. Any truly critical assessment of technology in a practice discipline such as nursing demands appraisal of its role in knowledge development and representation. Moreover, different technologies entail different human-machine relations that can be explored for their impact on what and how nurses know.

For example, computerized information systems in nursing may fail to capture and represent nursing practice adequately, and therefore may serve only to reinforce the invisibility of nursing work (e.g., Harney, 1993). Surveillance technologies, such as the varieties of machine monitoring, and prosthetic technologies, such as the varieties of organ transplantation techniques, can engender important changes in nursing constructions of the person and of health, which, in turn, may influence nursing practice. Such technologies make the very concepts of "person" and "health" dynamic ones, subject to rapid change. Technology has already transformed the brain-dead patient into a potential organ donor (Wolf, 1991) and childbearing into a pathogenic process (Davis-Floyd, 1992).

Technology is an essential component of nursing praxis, constituting thoughtful action in several realms of meaning. In nursing, it is a pervasive way of knowing our patients and their worlds that can cause us to forget how much of our knowing it has influenced. Technology is a way of knowing that can paradoxically "make us forget ourselves" (Reiser, 1984, p. 18).

REFERENCES

Abbey, J. C. (1978). Bioinstrumentation: Twentieth century slave. *Nursing Clinics of North America, 13,* 631-640.

Bean, M. A., Krahn, F. A., Anderson, B. L., & Yoshida, M. T. (1963). Monitoring patients through electronics. *American Journal of Nursing, 63,* 65-69.

Benner, P. (1984). *From novice to expert: Excellence and power in clinical nursing practice.* Menlo Park, CA: Addison-Wesley.

Brown, B. (1985). From the editor. *Nursing Administration Quarterly, 9,* iv-v.

Buber, M. (1958). *I and thou.* New York: Charles Scribner's Sons.

Bush, C. G. (1983). Women and the assessment of technology: To think, to be, to unthink, to free. In J. Rothschild (Ed.), *Machina ex dea: Feminist perspectives on technology* (pp. 151-170). New York: Pergamon.

Carper, B. (1978). Fundamental patterns of knowing in nursing. *Advances in Nursing Science, 1,* 13-23.

Channell, D. F. (1991). *The vital machine: A study of technology and organic life.* New York: Oxford University Press.

Cheek, J., & Rudge, T. (1994). Nursing as textually mediated reality. *Nursing Inquiry, 1,* 15-22.

Chinn, P. L. (1989). Nursing patterns of knowing and feminist thought. *Nursing and Health Care, 10,* 71-75.

Chinn, P. L., & Watson, J. (Eds.). (1994). *Art and aesthetics in nursing.* New York: National League for Nursing.

Cowan, R. S. (1983). *More work for mother: The ironies of household technology from the open hearth to the microwave.* New York: Basic Books.

Daffos, F. (1989). Access to the other patient. *Seminars in Perinatology, 13,* 252-259.

Davis-Floyd, R. E. (1992). *Birth as an American rite of passage.* Berkeley: University of California Press.

Dickoff, J., & James, P. (1992a). Highly technical but yet not impure: Varieties of basic knowledge. In L. H. Nicolls (Ed.), *Perspectives on nursing theory* (2nd ed., pp. 572-575). Philadelphia: J. B. Lippincott.

Dickoff, J., & James, P. (1992b). Taking concepts as guides to action: Exploring kinds of know-how. In L. H. Nicolls (Ed.), *Perspectives on nursing theory* (2nd ed., pp. 576-580). Philadelphia: J. B. Lippincott.

Duden, B. (1993). *Disembodying women: Perspectives on pregnancy and the unborn.* Cambridge, MA: Harvard University Press.

Fairman, J. (1992). Watchful vigilance: Nursing care, technology, and the development of intensive care units. *Nursing Research, 41,* 56-60.

Faulkner, W. (1994). Conceptualizing knowledge used in innovation: A second look at the science-technology distinction and industrial innovation. *Science, Technology, and Human Values, 19,* 425-458.

Ferguson, E. S. (1977). The mind's eye: Nonverbal thought in technology. *Science, 197,* 827-836.

Fletcher, J. F. (1988). *The ethics of genetic control: Ending reproductive roulette.* Buffalo, NY: Prometheus.

Harding, S. (1991). *Whose science? Whose knowledge? Thinking from women's lives.* Ithaca, NY: Cornell University Press.

Harney, M. (1993). Computation and gender. *Research in Philosophy and Technology, 13,* 57-71.

Ihde, D. (1979). *Technics and praxis.* Boston: Kluwer.

Ihde, D. (1983). *Existential technics.* Albany: State University of New York Press.

Ihde, D. (1990). *Technology and the lifeworld: From garden to earth.* Bloomington: Indiana University Press.

Ihde, D. (1991). *Instrumental realism: The interface between philosophy of science and philosophy of technology.* Bloomington: Indiana University Press.

Ingold, T. (1988). Tools, minds and machines: An excursion in the philosophy of technology. *Techniques et culture, 12,* 151-176.

Jacobs-Kramer, M. K., & Chinn, P. L. (1988). Perspectives on knowing: A model of nursing knowledge. *Scholarly Inquiry for Nursing Practice, 2,* 129-139.

Johnson, J. L. (1994). A dialectical examination of nursing art. *Advances in Nursing Science, 17*(1), 1-14.

Jonas, H. (1979). Toward a philosophy of technology. *Hastings Center Report, 9,* 34-43.

Katims, I. (1993). Nursing as aesthetic experience and the notion of practice. *Scholarly Inquiry for Nursing Practice, 7,* 269-278.

Layton, E. (1974). Technology as knowledge. *Technology and Culture, 15,* 31-41.

Lynch, M., & Woolgar, S. (Eds.). (1988). *Representation in scientific practice.* Boston: Kluwer Academic.

Machines in perspective (Special feature). (1965). *American Journal of Nursing, 65,* 67-85.

Mattingly, S. S. (1992). The maternal-fetal dyad: Exploring the two-patient obstetric model. *Hastings Center Report, 22,* 13-18.

Melosh, B. (1982). *"The physician's hand": Work culture and conflict in American nursing.* Philadelphia: Temple University Press.

Minckley, B. B. (1968). The multiphasic human-to-human monitor (ICU model): Nursing observation in the intensive care unit. *Nursing Clinics of North America, 3,* 29-39.

Mitcham, C. (1994). *Thinking through technology: The path between engineering and philosophy.* Chicago: University of Chicago Press.

Petchesky, R. P. (1987). Fetal images: The power of visual culture in the politics of reproduction. In M. Stanworth (Ed.), *Reproductive technologies: Gender, motherhood, and medicine* (pp. 57-80). Minneapolis: University of Minnesota Press.

Phenix, P. H. (1964). *Realms of meaning.* New York: McGraw-Hill.

Reiser, S. J. (1984). The machine at the bedside: Technological transformations of practices and values. In S. J. Reiser & M. Anbar (Eds.), *The machine at the bedside: Strategies for using technology in patient care* (pp. 3-19). Cambridge, UK: Cambridge University Press.

Rorty, R. (1979). *Philosophy and the mirror of nature.* Princeton, NJ: Princeton University Press.

Rothenberg, D. (1993). *Hand's end: Technology and the limits of nature.* Berkeley: University of California Press.

Sandelowski, M. (1988). A case of conflicting paradigms: Nursing and reproductive technology. *Advances in Nursing Science, 10*(3), 35-45.

Sandelowski, M. (1994a). Channel of desire: Fetal ultrasonography in two use-contexts. *Qualitative Health Research, 4,* 262-280.

Sandelowski, M. (1994b). Separate but less unequal: Ultrasonography and the transformation of expectant mother/fatherhood. *Gender & Society, 8,* 230-245.

Sandelowski, M., & Black, B. P. (1994). The epistemology of expectant parenthood. *Western Journal of Nursing Research, 16,* 601-614.

Stafford, B. M. (1993). Voyeur or observer? Enlightenment thoughts on the dilemmas of display. *Configurations: Journal of Literature, Science, and Technology, 1,* 95-128.

Starkman, M. N. (1976). Psychological responses to the use of the fetal monitor during labor. *Psychosomatic Medicine, 38,* 269-277.

Tisdale, S. (1986). Swept away by technology. *American Journal of Nursing, 86,* 429-430.

Wagner, D. (1980). The proletarianization of nursing in the United States, 1932-1946. *International Journal of Health Services, 10,* 271-290.

Wajcman, J. (1991). *Feminism confronts technology.* University Park: Pennsylvania State University Press.

Weeks, S. L. (1988). *"She's a bargain at any price": The effect of technology on hospital nursing.* Unpublished doctoral dissertation, Washington State University, Pullman.

White, J. (1995). Patterns of knowing: Review, critique, and update. *Advances in Nursing Science, 17*(4), 73-86.

White, L. (1962). *Medieval technology and social change.* Oxford, UK: Oxford University Press.

Wiener, C., Strauss, A., Fagerhaugh, S., & Suczek, B. (1979). Trajectories, biographies and the evolving medical technology scene: Labor and delivery and the intensive care nursery. *Sociology of Health and Illness, 1,* 261-283.

Wolf, Z. R. (1986). *Nurses' work: The sacred and the profane.* Philadelphia: University of Pennsylvania Press.

Wolf, Z. R. (1991). Nurses' experiences giving postmortem care to patients who have donated organs: A phenomenological study. *Scholarly Inquiry for Nursing Practice, 5,* 73-87.

Wolfer, J. (1993). Aspects of "reality" and ways of knowing in nursing: In search of an integrating paradigm. *Image: The Journal of Nursing Scholarship, 25,* 141-146.

PART II

Applied Theoretical Knowledge

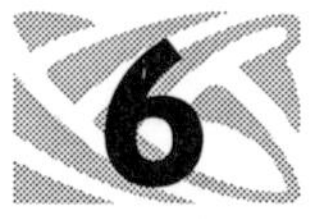

Enlightenment in Nursing

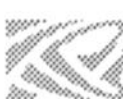

DONNA M. TRAINOR

As discussed in this chapter, *enlightenment* refers to a form of questioning that assures the ongoing generation of new knowledge. This form of questioning assumes that the autonomy inherent in professional practice extends as well to the inquiry based upon that practice. Through a historical review targeting the impact of social systems related to the development of nursing practice and nursing education, this chapter transgresses those assumptive barriers that preclude a sustained enlightenment and prevent the establishment of nursing's authority within a social environment.

Enlightenment as a philosophical movement of the eighteenth century was characterized by a lively questioning of authority. It was a particular posture of inquiry toward the nature of authority as pertains to reason. This philosophical inquiry was not a means to an end in the sense of providing a polling of opinion for ultimately accepting or rejecting an existing authority. Rather, inquiry was an end in itself that targeted authority as the context for formulating questions to assure the generation of new knowledge. It was a vehicle for providing critical knowledge regarding the nature of authority.

Authority, in the sense that it was understood in the Enlightenment, was cast in the broadest of terms. It was synonymous with the maker, the creator, the originator, as in one who composes a book or a musical score. Authority today, by comparison, is commonly understood as government or command or one who generates opinions, supports opinions, or is empowered to govern or command due to opinion. According to Kant, writing in the late eighteenth century, enlightenment means an exit from immaturity (Foucault, 1984). As examples, he asserts that maturity is being reached when understanding replaces a book or when conscience takes the place of a priest. Enlightenment is a process in which we collectively participate as a voluntary act of personal courage to know.

As for authority in the practice of nursing, it is the common sense of the profession that the route of knowledge in approaching enlightenment or reaching maturity lies in being professional. In this sense, the profession trusts that the autonomy issued by the provider is sufficient to assure both the preservation and the evolution of the profession. Autonomy is a quality displayed in individual self-regulating activity that renders that activity independent and the agent of that activity accountable. Autonomy in nursing implies activity regulated by the profession as an aggregate and/or by the individual professional. Understanding autonomy as authority sets a relationship between autonomy conceived as authority and the social systems that collectively serve as an environmental context for authority. Nursing operates as a profession within the context of social systems of education and health care. Nursing assumes its authority in education and aspires to establish its authority in health care. Nursing has traditionally functioned within the context of the health care system, yet the profession has not situated authority within the context of health care as a social system.

Whatever contemporary issues in health care there are, they undoubtedly have impacts upon what it is to be professional. Resolution of these issues leads to the delegation of who provides care, decisions as to how care is provided, and the delimiting of the context for the provision of care. Calling to task the meaning of autonomous practice and formulating the question, What is enlightenment in nursing? assures provider participation in shaping these resolutions. An investigation of the function of self-regulating activity as the hallmark of autonomous practice is essential to the preservation of nursing and key to its evolution. Such investigation is crucial to the ongoing generation of new knowledge as an essential premise of evolution. Donahue (1991) notes, "Nursing knowledge is one area in particular in which nurses worldwide are constantly seeking to clarify its distinctiveness in order that the nursing knowledge base being developed provides unity for the profession" (p. 326). The unity of which Donahue speaks assures collective participation. The chapters in Kikuchi and Simmons's (1992) edited volume examine the significance and scope of philosophical inquiry in nursing and identify as problematic the disproportional lack of formal philosophical inquiry among nursing scholars compared with other areas of interest. Although philosophical inquiry has grown in the past few years, nurse scholars more commonly question phenomena encountered in practice than the nature of practice itself as a phenomenon. Investigating the nature of autonomous practice is prerequisite to questioning the nature of enlightenment in nursing, clarifying the distinctiveness of nursing knowledge, and identifying nursing questions.

As a profession, nursing represents collective participation that engenders a particular structure of knowledge. It approaches maturity when nursing care is provided without prescription and when primary health care needs are addressed despite place or agency. The route to maturity is individual autonomous practice. The individual practitioner as authority is proactive and not reliant upon direction from sources outside the profession. This maturity is characterized as the act of personal courage to know. In this sense, the professional participates collectively in determining what nursing is and how nursing is practiced. The questions to be addressed in this chapter are three: What is enlightenment in nursing? What barriers currently operate in attaining enlightenment? What are the conditions necessary for the possibility of a sustained enlightenment?

WHAT IS ENLIGHTENMENT IN NURSING?

An investigation of authority consistent with the way it was understood during the Enlightenment presumes an established relationship among such concepts as self-regulation, knowledge, and activity.

Piagetian philosophy, epigenetic epistemology, provides a comprehensive system of thought addressing self-regulatory mechanisms as they pertain to knowledge and activity as phenomena. This philosophy is cast within the language of biology and its principles. In *Biology and Knowledge: An Essay on the Relations Between Organic Regulations and Cognitive Processes,* Piaget (1971) distinguishes two types of regulatory mechanisms: One regulates structure and the other regulates function. The mere possibility of differing types of self-regulating mechanisms is of particular interest in the study of nursing activity, as it speaks to alternatives in defining its function. The differences apparent in comparing these types of mechanisms pertain directly to the nature of nursing's knowledge structure, the function of its activity, and the designation of the phenomenon it questions. An analysis of these two mechanisms leads to the identification of principles of self-regulation and assists in the critical evaluation of the nature of autonomy conceived as authority.

Piaget's examination of these mechanisms has impacts upon both the structure of knowledge and the function of that structure in the ongoing acquisition of knowledge. According to Piaget, structural self-regulating mechanisms, such as homeorhesis, promote a dynamic equilibrium, whereas functional self-regulatory mechanisms, such as homeostasis, sustain a static equilibrium. Both mechanisms are tied to environment. Functional self-regulating mechanisms achieve stability by insulating toward a static equilibrium in response to changes initiated in the environment. Structural self-regulating mechanisms achieve a dynamic equilibrium through evolution with the environment. In the first type, functional self-regulation, change is predicated as contingent upon the environment, whereas in the second, structural self-regulation, change incorporates the environment as essential to the evolution of the structure. Change occurs in one as passive resistance; in the other, change occurs through active participation. In the former, change is governed externally. In the latter, change is self-governed. The authority of individual providers in nursing presupposes individual activity operating with the social environment but independent of recourse to an environmental social system as agent in governing change. The self-regulatory mechanisms identified by Piaget and implied in autonomous activity must be structural in nature to assure authority connoting self-governance. If the profession inadvertently defines its activity consistent with what Piaget identifies as a functional self-regulating mechanism, then the authority inherent in autonomy, as a value, collapses.

Piaget's interest in this distinction is shared by psychologist Gordon Allport (1955), who targets autonomy as a concept central to his personality theory. The distinction Allport makes involves two levels of a core concept called *functional autonomy.* The first, preservative functional autonomy, Allport sees as illustrating infrahuman preservative activities or circular mechanisms that keep the organism going. The second, propriate functional autonomy, refers to acquired interests in attainment of progressively higher levels of authentic maturity. The clear parallel between Piaget's notion of two types of self-regulating mechanisms and Allport's notion of two levels of functional autonomy is the characterization of activity as a dynamic interchange between the organism and the environment. Professional practice must be couched in such a form of dynamic activity if knowledge generated through practice is to serve authority authentically in guiding the selection of phenomena determined appropriate to research.

In an essay on the nature of knowledge titled "What Is Enlightenment?" Foucault (1984) discusses the function of authority within the context of inquiry and identifies assumptions essential to formulating questions that yield new knowledge. The principles inherent in the distinctions made by Piaget and Allport point to a set of assumptions that fit as an assumptive base supporting the nature of contemporary inquiry as portrayed by Foucault (1984):

> Today when a periodical asks its readers a question, it does so in order to collect opinions on some subject about which everyone has an opinion already; there is not much likelihood of learning anything new. In the eighteenth century, editors preferred to question the public on problems that did not yet have solutions. (p. 32)

Allport's preservative functional autonomy and Piaget's functional self-regulatory mechanism point to a static, circulatory activity that, envisioned as dialogue, serves only to sustain inquiry; activity so conceived cannot advance a dialogue that evolves as a discourse for inquiry assuring the generation of new knowledge. Authority must interact with the social context to initiate new knowledge. Eighteenth-century inquiry, compared with that of today, was of a different order, an order that, in contrast, seemed to presume the assumptions implied in the dynamic concepts of propriate functional autonomy and structural self-regulating mechanisms. This earlier form of inquiry calls forth the authority that, by today's standards, arrogantly expresses itself in the voluntary act of personal courage to know.

Enlightenment in nursing presupposes philosophical agreement between the individual professional and the aggregate in their joint responsibility of regulating practice. In his text *Cosmopolis,* Toulmin (1990) addresses the significance of the individual and the collective within the context of eighteenth-century thought. Toulmin notes that eighteenth-century inquiry was adopted as a worldview precisely because the questions asked and the solutions put forth were, for the most part, of a scope that appealed to a collective participation and the hidden agenda of the members of that collective. Such inquiry was irresistible, both in inviting individual interest and in captivating the individual's personal courage to know. According to Toulmin, in this way, the power of inquiry is attributed to the adoption of Enlightenment as a worldview. Foucault's essay "What Is Enlightenment?" (1984) advances the view that enlightenment is, in effect, a form of inquiry; to be enlightened is to question in a particular way. This form of inquiry represents an ongoing commencement of formulating new questions, never a conclusion that confirms or maintains an existing level of thought through a polling of opinion. Enlightenment symbolizes a solution that serves as a question of its own design, not a response to a question as given, limited in its relevance to the particular instance. Foucault claims that enlightenment articulates something new from what has yet to be questioned, not an opinion on what is presumed unquestionable. Enlightenment serves as a particular posture of inquiry. Although it may provoke a solution, it is never aimed at resolution.

The question, What is enlightenment in nursing? is appropriately posed as a problem that does not yet have a solution. To pose the question is to invite enlightenment in nursing. Questioning the nature of authority in practice questions the nature of autonomy. Such inquiry promotes understanding of the role that authority subsumes in the generation of new knowledge. Structural self-regulating knowledge is enlightened knowledge. It involves inquiry as a dynamic interactivity between the profession as a collective and the agents of such social systems that otherwise potentially compromise social environment as the context of practice. Autonomous practice in nursing is jeopardized if sources external to the profession prompt a distortion of nursing's unique commitment to society by engaging the profession in commentary responding to questions that fixate the profession. As a matter of assumption, if the initiative for change originates in external sources, then these sources are authorized to govern practice.

WHAT BARRIERS CURRENTLY OPERATE IN ATTAINING ENLIGHTENMENT?

In examining the barriers that operate in attaining enlightenment, I am limited in this chapter to an exploration of those circumstances or conditions that may have contributed to the profession's inadvertently adopting a sustained connotation of autonomy that is inconsistent with autonomy conceived as authority. Given Piaget's description of functional self-regulating mechanisms and Allport's definition of preservative functional autonomy, can a set of circumstances or conditions be identified that fostered this particular adoption and that prevails today, operating as a barrier to inquiry directed at the nature of autonomy? The tenacity of such a set of circumstances in deterring enlightenment would, no doubt, be of the order described by Toulmin in its appeal to a collective participation and the hidden agenda of the members of that collective. Is nursing idiosyncratic both as a profession and a discipline in that its knowledge structure is identical to and at one with the function of knowledge in the activity of that profession? Does this unique configuration of nursing's disciplinary knowledge structure and function prompt a hidden agenda that predisposes the profession to the effect of a particular set of circumstances or conditions?

Foucault's method of inquiry, characterized as archaeology of knowledge, serves as an approach to a historical exploration of the development of nursing as a discipline. Perhaps the profession's collective adoption of what Allport terms functional autonomy is to date unquestioned precisely because the conditions that affected that particular adoption serve specifically to insulate against such inquiry. For Foucault, Allport's functional autonomy typifies contemporary inquiry. The generation of knowledge reflected in nursing periodicals is, in effect, overwhelmingly characteristic of contemporary inquiry. Judging from what is published, nursing inquiry largely seeks commentary on issues through a polling of opinion. It would be curious to consider, in light of Foucault's thesis, what the possible complexion of nursing literature might be if manuscripts accepted for publication needed to qualify as new knowledge and manuscripts written in response to those of others necessarily were characterized as editorials.

Walsh notes the benefit of historical review in his *Philosophy of History* (1967). He claims, "The first aim of the historian, when he is asked to explain some event or another, is to see it as part of such a process, to locate it in its context by mentioning other events with which it is bound up" (pp. 24-25). The historical review is consistent with Foucault's archaeological method. The impact of learning and knowing as concepts in the developmental history of nursing is indeed peculiar. To understand how the structure and function of nursing knowledge are affected by history, we must investigate the impact of education as a social system on authority. The development of collegiate nursing and the development of behavioristic psychology are bound up as events both in time and in place. The relationship between these events provides, in part, an explanation for how it is that nursing, to date, has resisted inquiry aimed at either questioning activity as learned behavior or questioning activity as praxis or know-how based upon autonomy. Nursing's unique configuration, in the inseparability of its disciplinary structure and its professional function, accounts for a predisposition and vulnerability to behaviorism.

In the early twentieth century, the first systematic study of learned behavior was introduced by behaviorist John B. Watson (1930). The philosophical assumptions of behaviorism served as a panacea for the troubles of a Western world enveloped in the Great Depression that began in 1929. Behaviorism, as a perspective, was totally in concert with the spirit of the times and the assumptive factors that targeted learning as the central category of behaviorism and guaranteed the influence of the environment to be writ large. At this time, nursing was emerging as an academic discipline. The appeal of behaviorism to nursing as a collective and to the hidden agenda of its participant members was no less a driving force than was the general appeal of behaviorism, as evidenced in its coloring of all of Western societal systems. That this influence is sustained in nursing as artifact is a tribute to the unique configuration of the discipline.

Nursing education and nursing practice historically share a common place or environment and a related common philosophical base that together represent an underlying model for practice. In the early twentieth century, nursing educators urged the relocation of the education of professional nurses from the clinic to the academy. In moving from the clinic to the academy, collegiate nursing educators tacitly assumed that the separation of nursing from the service environment and its related philosophy of practice assured the invocation of a new philosophy for the profession. The timing was impeccable, and the place or environment was the common ground. The pervasive effects and profound implications of behaviorism as a movement upon the development of nursing are crucial. The relationship between these events can be shown to account, in part, for a prevailing synthetic separation of the function of practice from the structure of knowledge in nursing. Understanding the commonality of assumptions that existed at that point in time leads to the identification of specific barriers that no doubt operate insidiously to deter enlightenment in nursing. Consistent with the reigning philosophical perspective of behaviorism, it was reasonable to assume that a different environment was sufficient cause to support an epistemological distinction between professional and technical educational preparation. Subsequently, the profession of nursing has proceeded while constrained by the epistemological limitations and accompanying philosophical implications of a behaviorist position grounded in logical positivism. Within the context of the behaviorist school perspective, a perspective that predominated in both American thought and Western society from the early 1920s through the mid-1950s, an environmental "switch" could singularly provide sufficient reason for concluding "professional" behavior had been established for nursing.

Unexamined, this set of assumptions implicitly operates to limit the developing knowledge base of nursing by constraining the phenomena considered appropriate to nursing research in deference to actual practice. As a perspective, behaviorism is antithetical to cognitivism, and at an assumptive level, it precludes the possibility of an epistemology for nursing. From the standpoint of authority as it relates to education as a social system, this led to the adoption of a set of assumptions as a faulty premise that suppresses motivation in the area of philosophical inquiry in nursing and deters scholarly efforts in the area of qualitatively distinguishing professional and technical education in nursing. Scholarly efforts that are undertaken, as a philosophical search for what is retrospectively recognized as epistemological autonomy, are impeded by the tautology embedded in the assumptions of their very inspiration. The set of assumptions directly attributable to the physical division of collegiate nursing from the clinic now serve to impede the very outcome that was its raison d'être—the generation of a distinct knowledge base for professional nursing.

The designation of the practice of nursing framed in behavioral assumptions is unquestionable from the perspective of authority in nursing. To the extent that nursing scholars attempt to develop a distinct epistemological base, the implicit assumptive base of behaviorism philosophically limits that development in that (a) it presupposes that the generation of nursing knowledge is determined exclusively by the general purview of the academy as an environment, and (b) it fails to oblige academe to define nursing knowledge in terms of praxis, as praxis in nursing has been assumed to be determined by the clinical environment, namely, client care outcomes as dependent variables for evaluating educational interventions (Smith, 1979). Lack of philosophical exploration of the assumptions inherent in this supposed distinction consequently serves to fortify an existing "hospital school" identification of nursing activity as behavior subject to the contingencies of its environment. The machinations of the early "training" model of nursing education known to all remind us of the determinants that designated the "place" where the student nurse would *learn* her place and *behave* professionally as a direct response of unquestioning compliance with elaborate rule structures that governed the environment that was nursing education. This identification of nursing activity as behavior was implicitly transferred with the relocation of "professional nursing" to the collegiate environment.

The presuppositions implied in the continued use of environment or place as a concept central to the practice of nursing sustain a recalcitrance to agree upon a common philosophical base that would serve to distinguish technical and professional nursing and, concurrently, to advance a shared epistemological base for practice. The continued prominence of place in differentiating practice presupposes that the activity of nursing is environmentally contingent. From an academic perspective, according to Bevis (1993), "investing behaviorist theory with exclusive theoretical credibility has enabled it to affect nursing education and practice both in positive and in restrictive ways. . . . Restrictiveness, oppression and categorization of human beings as objects was unforeseen and a long unrecognized outcome of behaviorism" (p. 57). Griffin (1980) notes:

> An extensive (first philosophical and then more general) literature criticizing the objectives approach to understanding curriculum design has been available for some years. . . . (The objectives approach is junior, though pretentious, relation of the systems approach coming from the same mechanistic and behavioristic stable.) . . . The criticisms, most unfortunately, appear less well-known than early influential statements such as Bloom's Taxonomy of Educational Objectives, conceived on a behaviorist model. Despite the fact that the taxonomy is too full of epistemological and other serious errors to be worth patching up . . . the taxonomy retains a remarkable grip over (at least) syllabus construction. (pp. 270-271)

From a contemporary perspective, environment is key to characteristically distinguishing professional education from nonprofessional or technical education. Consider the array of nursing education models that have developed over time—each model has a different approach for license preparation and each is distinguished by its particular environmental characteristics. Today, each continues to be represented; each, respectively, produces a nurse whose distinction in practice is judged solely on the basis of behavior defined within the constraints of a clinical environment. The result typifies a profession fixated, a profession restrained in its evolution through its own proliferation. It is a profession and discipline ironically constrained by an autonomy characterized by functional regulation. Autonomy, so characterized, connotes independence while operating to assure dependence to environmental contingencies by sustaining a static equilibrium that behaves in response to change initiated in the environment. In *Behavior and Evolution,* Piaget (1978) succinctly addresses the phenomenon of such a relationship:

> Where physiological assimilation proceeds by simple repetition, without reference to earlier phases, behavioral assimilation engenders a memory which increases the number of relationships and thus contributes to its own extension. As far as accommodations imposed by external variations which modify assimilation in varying degrees, these are merely suffered passively by the physiological organization and result only in replacements, always kept to a minimum, of particular aspects of an assimilatory cycle. (pp. 141-142)

If nursing education is, by analogy, considered as the "physiological organization" in this instance, then reflective philosophical inquiry serves as a vehicle of "reference to earlier phases" and a conduit for effecting evolution through transformation. Without such inquiry, nursing suffers passively in response to external efforts at change and generates its own replacements in the absence of transformation.

WHAT ARE THE CONDITIONS NECESSARY FOR THE POSSIBILITY OF A SUSTAINED ENLIGHTENMENT?

This chapter questions the nature of autonomous practice in nursing, using a form of inquiry characteristic of the Enlightenment. Through this inquiry the residual affects of behaviorism are identified as a barrier specifically operating against the generation of new knowledge. Nursing's inability to establish authority as autonomy is attributed to the effects of behaviorism in subverting the formulation of questions that generate new knowledge. The question posed in this chapter and the method of inquiry displayed in formulating that question set the stage for sustaining enlightenment. Enlightenment will be typified by ongoing inquiry where questions ask for solutions that do not yet exist, questions irresistible to the personal courage to know. The formulation of these questions calls for a search that seeks inconsistency, dissonance, and discrepancy as markers of assumptions that serve as fertile ground in the generation of new knowledge. The aim is not to resolve the inconsistency or to reduce the essential tension of the dissonance, but to identify and transgress the assumptive barriers themselves. In nursing, disparity exists between knowledge and the application of knowledge; exploration of the assumptions that give rise to that disparity lead to the generation of new knowledge.

For example, Kuhn demonstrates, in *The Structure of Scientific Revolutions* (1962), that how science is practiced is different from how scientists say they practice science. Kuhn's thesis—which, incidentally, uses Piagetian assumptions as an organizational device—is implicated in the identification of practical knowledge in nursing. In *From Novice to Expert,* Benner (1984) notes the significance of Kuhn's thesis in the identification and description of clinical knowledge. Drawing from the compendium of exemplars she has compiled, Benner claims in effect that what nurses say they do in practice is not what they do as practice. Those who teach and practice repeatedly report incompatibility and lack of agreement between the two. Benner's project is devoted to explicating the clinical knowledge inherent in this inconsistency; in this chapter my aim is to question the barriers to enlightenment that promote such inconsistency. Benner (1984) attributes to Kuhn (1977) the value of a hermeneutic approach in achieving understandings of clinical knowledge, quoting advice Kuhn gives to his students that serves by inference to focus upon the nature of inconsistency between knowledge and the application of knowledge:

> When reading the works of an important thinker, look first for the apparent absurdities in the text and ask yourself how a sensible person could have written them. When you find an answer, I continue, when you find those passages make sense, then you may find that more central passages, ones you previously thought you understood, have changed their meaning. (Kuhn, 1977, pp. xi-xii)

In his own work and in the instruction of his students, Kuhn deliberately searches for texts and materials that evidence inconsistency, dissonance, and discrepancy as the basis of transgressing assumptions that otherwise operate against the learning of anything new.

Piaget's (1971) distinction regarding self-regulatory mechanisms identifies the source of disagreement between knowledge and autonomous practice by making explicit the disparity between the two. His thesis assumes that activity is inseparable from the nature of knowledge. What *nursing says* it does as nursing assumes this inseparability. This is important, as the difference between the activity of nursing as functionally regulated as behavior and the activity of nursing as structurally self-regulated as praxis characterizes nursing knowledge as enlightened. Praxis incorporates what is known as nursing with what one knows how to do as nursing. Praxis supplants skills of practice with strategies of practice. Behavior is learned; praxis presupposes know-how by the provider as autonomous authority. This distinction is a distinction between learning or conditioning and knowledge or cognition. Viewed solely from the standpoint of outcome, the difference between the two is subtle. The difference becomes crucial, however, when viewed both at an assumptive level and at the level of implications, if, as Foucault (1984) claims, there is a "likelihood of learning anything new" (p. 32).

Targeting autonomy as the basis for authority in nursing serves as a point of departure for formulating questions that assure the generation of new knowledge. What is enlightenment in nursing? There is not yet a solution. Viewed as an end in itself, inquiry assumes a posture that justifies the means for an exit from immaturity. This is the point of departure suggested here. To suggest a conclusion is anathema to whatever it may ultimately mean to be enlightened.

Central to the activity of philosophizing is the notion of a search; to search philosophically is to unearth those belief systems that operate insidiously to shape and potentially determine the metaphysics, epistemology, ethics, and aesthetics of disciplinary thought. For Foucault, the philosophical search is just that (Gutting, 1989); it is not a forecast of what should be the case, and it never serves as a resolution. Foucault characterizes this line of inquiry as an epistemological unearthing or archaeology of knowledge. This method as an activity is synonymous with the will to truth, providing those within the discipline and its system of thought the opportunity to transgress the boundary conditions of itself as a society. If serious scholarly effort in the activity of philosophical inquiry is to be effective in articulating a formal philosophical base to which the profession can collectively subscribe, we must, as individuals, philosophically search for and identify the fundamental assumptions from which nursing currently operates. This chapter is intended to initiate and stimulate such an enterprise.

When Foucault suggests that knowledge is power, he suggests that power is vested in the authority of enlightenment and that the generation of new knowledge that characterizes enlightenment occurs in the transgression of global boundaries through compliance with local regulation. This is not to say that it is a simple matter to ask a question for which there is not yet an answer, nor is it to suggest that to formulate such a question will assure new knowledge. It is to say that new knowledge is possible only through inquiry directed at authority. This is not to question authority by enjoining commentary in its contemporary interpretation as one who generates or supports opinions or is empowered to govern or command due to opinion; rather, it is to question authority as the maker, the creator, the originator, as in one who composes a book or a musical score. To question authority in this sense is to make recourse to history. As Foucault writes in *Discipline and Punish* (1979), "I would like to write history. Why? Simply because I am interested in the Past? No, if one means by that writing a history of the past in terms of the present. Yes, if one means writing the history of the present" (pp. 30-31). In a most contemporary sense, to formulate such a question is to understand what is at stake when Foucault addresses the relationship between power (i.e., authority) and knowledge.

REFERENCES

Allport, G. (1955). *Becoming.* London: Yale University Press.

Benner, P. (1984). *From novice to expert: Excellence and power in clinical nursing practice.* Menlo Park, CA: Addison-Wesley.

Bevis, E. O. (1993). Alliances for destiny: Education and practice. *Nursing Management, 24,* 56-61.

Donahue, M. P. (1991). Inquiry, insight and history: Philosophy in a nurse's world. *Journal of Professional Nursing, 7,* 326.

Foucault, M. (1979). *Discipline and punish: The birth of the prison* (2nd ed.). New York: Vintage.

Foucault, M. (1984). *The Foucault reader* (P. Rabinow, Ed.). New York: Pantheon.

Griffin, A. P. (1980). Philosophy and nursing. *Journal of Advanced Nursing, 5,* 261-272.

Gutting, G. (1989). *Michel Foucault's archaeology of scientific reason.* Cambridge, UK: Cambridge University Press.

Kikuchi, J. F., & Simmons, H. (Eds.). (1992). *Philosophic inquiry in nursing.* Newbury Park, CA: Sage.

Kuhn, T. S. (1962). *The structure of scientific revolutions.* Chicago: University of Chicago Press.

Kuhn, T. S. (1977). *The essential tension.* Chicago: University of Chicago Press.

Piaget, J. (1971). *Biology and knowledge: An essay on the relations between organic regulations and cognitive processes.* Chicago: University of Chicago Press.

Piaget, J. (1978). *Behavior and evolution.* New York: Random House.

Smith, J. P. (1979). Is the nursing profession really research-based? *Journal of Advanced Nursing, 4,* 319-325.

Toulmin, S. (1990). *Cosmopolis: The hidden agenda of modernity.* New York: Free Press.

Walsh, W. H. (1967). *Philosophy of history.* New York: Harper Torchbooks.

Watson, J. B. (1930). *Behaviorism.* New York: W. W. Norton.

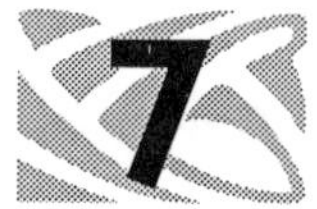

Implications of the Caring/Competence Dichotomy

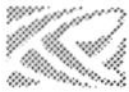

SIGRÍDUR HALLDÓRSDÓTTIR

Given our modern technological world, with its dehumanizing potential, the need for caring in nursing is unquestioned. It is imperative that nurses make a special effort to sustain a caring ideology. However, the artificial dichotomy between caring and competence that has emerged in some of the existing scholarly work is most unfortunate, given that nursing is a practical science in which competence is primary, especially from the patient's perspective. In this chapter, I explore this dichotomy and argue that, if we want to be truly progressive in nursing, the issue is not one of favoring either technology and competence or caring. To promote the art and science of nursing, we need both competence and caring; they are the essential ingredients of professional caring.

IN SEARCH OF EPISTEMOLOGY THAT IS TRUE TO NURSING

Through dialectical discussion, scientists are supposed to apprehend fundamental ideas (Oldroyd, 1989). For several years now, there has been discussion and debate within the nursing science literature on the nature of caring, competence, and technology in nursing, and the relationship of these to the philosophy of science in nursing. It appears that there is an urgent need for science that not only guides the logic of nursing practice but also forms a socially appropriate context for the evaluation of it. Bottorff (1991) has pointed out that "the practical science of nursing is that which defines the area of special competence of nurses, provides a legitimate basis for nursing's authority, and provides the methods for discovering and accumulating new knowledge for nursing" (p. 28). Whereas I view nursing as still in search of epistemology that is true to its practical science, some, including Rawnsley (1994), believe that such a paradigm already exists:

> Sometimes I wonder if it has occurred to anyone else that nursing does not have to shop in other disciplines to find a paradigm that fits. Nursing is, in itself, a paradigm. Nursing is an existential worldview, an essential human service in which the provider and the client are mutually shaped by professional values, societal change, and personal meaning. (p. 189)

Although there may be some truth in this, the questions posed over the past few decades still must be addressed. What is nursing? And what should its domain entail? I believe that we ought to confront the question of which defining characteristics of the discipline are worth preserving and which can be dismissed without substantive damage. Rawnsley (1994) asserts that, until now, the nurse-patient relationship has enjoyed protected status as a distinguishing characteristic of the discipline, representing the "conceptual cornerstone of its generational continuity of identity" (p. 186). The essence of nursing has been understood as "the caring connection that transcends time and culture" (p. 189). Although caring, including the "caring connection" between patient and nurse, is understood as a moral obligation for nursing, Bishop and Scudder (1996) and Morse, Bottorff, Neander, and Solberg (1991) remind us that it must be demonstrated and not simply proclaimed. If caring is to be the "central, and unifying feature of nursing," then it must be relevant to nursing practice and to the recipients of nursing care and not merely an internalized feeling on the part of the nurse. I believe, as Morse et al. (1991) seem to, that nursing loses legitimacy as a profession and as a discipline if caring has no behavioral requirement. If we content ourselves with a basically warmhearted, commonsense approach to caring as an essence of nursing, we may end up with idiosyncratic attitudes being accepted as legitimate answers to nursing problems and a sense that it is unnecessary to subject nursing practice to empirical tests of effectiveness (Bottorff, 1991). I agree with Clifford (1995) that most definitions of caring lack specificity and, without operational definitions and behavioral designations for caring, the scientific study of caring is limited. Finally, I side with Bottorff (1991), who further claims that "if caring cannot be shown to effect recovery from illness or enhance health in some way, the concept may not provide a useful foundation for the development of knowledge to guide nursing practice" (pp. 31-32).

Jones and Alexander (1993) point out that in nursing, technology and caring are commonly viewed as being at opposite ends of the philosophical spectrum—technology reflecting a mechanistic perspective and caring reflecting a humanistic perspective. As Locsin (1995) explains, the perception of technology and caring as dichotomous is so pervasive that "one who is technologically proficient may often be assumed to be incapable of expressing caring" (p. 201). According to Hawthorne and Yurkovich (1995), for example, "The professions have overemphasized the importance of science and technology which has consequently hampered their expression of caring, resulting in professionals who do not have a consensus about what they stand for and are unable to care about the people they serve" (p. 1087).

It is my assertion that emphasis on science and technology is not inherently bad; I believe that there need not be any causal relationship between such emphasis and lack of caring. The problem of "uncaring" is much more complex than the word implies. I recognize that technology can be a double-edged sword—while allowing nurses to intervene on behalf of patients and to extend human life, its use may at the same time diminish or degrade human dignity (Jones & Alexander, 1993). On the other hand, as we have come to depend upon technology both in society and in all health care delivery, it would be difficult for nurses to care for patients in its absence. As Locsin (1995) notes, machine technologies and caring in nursing need to be harmonious aspects of clinical nursing practice, and, indeed, health care. In the words of Gutierrez-Calleros (1992), the health professions need to "embrace and appreciate" art, science, and technology. A framework of nursing as caring should permit true technological competence in clinical nursing practice to be understood as an expression of caring (Bishop & Scudder, 1996; Locsin, 1995).

As such, technological competence assumes an indispensable place in contemporary clinical nursing practice. Ideally, it occurs "when machine technology is expressed competently while being grounded in the perspective of nursing as caring" (Locsin, 1995, p. 203). However, proficiency in machine technologies demonstrated without such grounding can emerge as technological competence devoid of a perception of people as human beings. It is only through the harmonious coexistence of machine technology and caring that the practice of nursing can be transformed into an experience of caring for the patient (Locsin, 1995). Although professionals and patients alike are grateful for the vast advances that have been achieved in medical and machine technology, it is vital that the use of such technology not compromise nurses' caring. Rather, "as nursing professionals become more and more technically adept, they will find new and improved ways to build strong, healing connections with patients" (Locsin, 1995, p. 203).

THE PATIENT'S PERSPECTIVE ON CARING AND COMPETENCE

As Bottorff (1991) points out, there seems to be a consensus within the nursing community that, for the most part, theorists have developed nurse-focused conceptualizations of caring. Jarrett and Payne (1995), for example, claim that there has been a general failure to take into account patients' perceptions of nurses, what patients wish to divulge to nurses, and how contextual and environmental factors may influence patients. These authors assert that "the focus of attention has been on what nurses are saying and doing during nurse-patient conversations and the patient has been largely ignored" (p. 77). Koch (1994) contends that the time has come for "negotiation-oriented evaluation" in nursing, in which all who are affected by the evaluation of a setting have a right to place their claims, concerns, and issues on the "negotiating table." This means that the participation of patients or recipients of nursing is central in the negotiation process. This view results in the emergence of the recipient as one of the central focuses of evaluation and thus quality assurance. Professional nursing roles necessarily involve practitioners' taking responsibility "to strive to become more effective and to seek valid feedback to ensure their actions are effective" (Johns, 1995, p. 28), which can "enable the development of practitioners' therapeutic potential to make a qualitative difference to people's lives, and in doing so, to enhance the societal value of nursing" (p. 29). Therefore, although what is termed as excellence in contemporary nursing will always have arbitrary elements (Käppeli, 1993), we can assume that it will include the condition of being patient-centered—that is, oriented toward the difference the nurse makes to a patient's quality of life.

In 1988, I completed a master's thesis on patients' perspectives of caring and uncaring encounters with nurses, in which I argue strongly for the importance of nurses' truly understanding their patients' perspectives (Halldórsdóttir, 1988, 1990). I became enchanted with the subject of the nursing recipient's perspective, and I have since completed nine studies, alone or with colleagues and students, with different groups of recipients regarding their perceptions of being patients and of caring and uncaring encounters with nurses and other health professionals (Halldórsdóttir, 1996). In each of these studies, my colleagues and I have considered the participants to be our co-researchers. As former recipients of nursing, the participants have emphasized competence as an essential component of professional caring. They have indicated that caring without competence was of little value to them as patients. For them, competence administered with caring was the ideal situation. In fact, they have argued that a nurse has to be both competent and caring to be truly professional. This "compassionate competence," as one participant called it, was summed up by another former patient in the following way:

> Competence is the most important thing. I mean you want to feel that whoever is looking after you knows what she or he is doing in terms of proper treatment. You don't want to get the wrong shots, you don't want too much, you don't want to be getting some oxygen where you should be getting something else. So, basically, that has to be taken care of, has to be taken for granted. So, the competence is number one, and if it's then administered with care then obviously you have an ideal situation.

So competence—and not only the appearance of competence, but legitimate competence—is an essential part of professional caring from the perspective of the recipient of nursing care. The nurse's acceptance of the importance of competence and of keeping skills up-to-date is therefore crucial, because nursing, like everything else, is ever changing.

At the same time, being professionally competent does not mean becoming less human. It is my contention that being truly professional in the health care field, or in any caring field, involves having the kind of knowledge and the kinds of skills that make up competence as well as the caring kind of attitude that many of my study participants have emphasized. Most of the former patients we have interviewed have been quite explicit about the importance of competence while at the same time emphasizing the human aspect of nursing care. One former patient illuminated the issue in the following way:

> If one wants to put it in a bit of a nutshell, the nurse has to stand on two legs. One is the professional side, and the other is the human side and the two of them have to belong to the same person. They have to be compatible. You can't have a professional side that is out of touch with the human side. And if those two are in harmony, as it were, belong to the other, I think a lot of the other things will follow.

As the preceding remarks show, patients do not see caring and competence as dichotomous; rather, they perceive them as two elements that have to go hand in hand to be of any value in professional caring. I have explored with some of my co-researchers whether caring and competence can in fact be segregated in nursing. This exploration is illustrated by the following dialogue:

R: Do you think we can differentiate between caring and competence?

C: Oh, I think you can, I mean if you talk about caring without competence it's pretty meaningless, but you would assume that the competence level is there . . . and then the caring is an essential added ingredient. . . .

R: So, the prerequisite would be the competence, but you would also have to have caring to be a good nurse?

C: Absolutely!

R: So, what would be your definition of caring, then?

C: Caring on its own doesn't mean much, I would imagine, I mean it has to be coupled with competence, I mean it's a profession! . . . Caring in itself is not good enough. . . .

R: Could we talk about professional caring? And then one aspect of that could be competence?

C: Well, the competence would be implied in the professional, I would imagine.

It is apparent that people who have been patients, or recipients of nursing care, see limited value in caring without competence. Some, however, have pointed out that the need for compassion and/or competence depends to an extent on the patient's situation. As one explained:

> If I was really ill, feeling miserable, feeling very bad, having a very rough time physically, at that point a nurse's competence is very, very important. But if I'm not feeling too bad, which has been mostly my case in the hospital—I mean I have had a lot of stays in the hospital which were a great amount of fun [laughs]—at that point I think I can accept an incompetent nurse more than I can accept an unnurturing nurse.

The accounts of the study participants demonstrate their perception of the importance of competence in professional caring. Many have emphasized, however, that competence alone often has limited value, as the following remarks illustrate:

> Well, I was thinking . . . the concrete things in your hospital stay are . . . you got bladder problems to deal with, or bowel problems, or diet or things like that, your medication, and your sleeping pills or whatever, those sorts of things. But the other thing that a patient is doing is a psychological thing. You're groping with the fact that, you know, that this is the third attack you have had of this disease, and what does that mean to my life? And that's very, very big. That's the other thing that is happening to that patient lying in that bed, and of course you don't see it. And a competent nurse who is not nurturing, or caring, whatever word we are using, is no help to me, you know. . . . The psychological trauma . . . competence doesn't help, there is no competence that can, unless by competence we are including this feature of caring or nurturing.

A professional caring approach includes genuine concern and respect for the individuality and well-being of the patient. The participants in my studies have explicitly emphasized that genuine concern for the patient as a person is one of the most important aspects of true professional caring. As one explained:

> I'm not referring to the mechanics of caring, but in genuinely wishing the patient well, that is, wishing the patient speedy recovery. I guess it's having those feelings, I mean it's more than just thinking, "Wouldn't it be nice if Mary Jones would be able to leave the hospital." It's a feeling tone. I say that because I'm suspicious that people pick up on the feeling tone, so if in fact you're indifferent and you just say that, you know, that he or she will be able to leave soon, it's nowhere near as effective and caring as if there really is genuine caring. So, it's a kind of a spiritual dimension to it, it's somehow that it matters, you know, it's almost tangible that it matters to someone that you graduate from the hospital, that you leave . . . upon your feet.

This and similar accounts indicate that the quality and the genuineness of the nurse's concern are perceived by the patient. It is not only *what* the nurse says and does that determines what the patient perceives as caring, but also *how* the nurse says and does things, and the feelings behind the nurse's words. When asked about the fundamental difference between caring and uncaring, one former patient elaborated:

> It seems to me primarily the quality of the intention, which is a hard thing to specify, you sort of, you feel it, and intuit it, I guess, or

> something like that, in the transaction. So it's not what's done, it's the way it's done or something like that. Or it's not even necessarily what's said, but the way that it's said. It might be the tone of voice, or sometimes it's the little extra efforts, you know, it's the plumping of pillows or just the moment for a kind word or just popping a head in the door and saying, "How are you doing? Is everything okay?" So, it can be little things like that, but often even just in the executing of routines, the bringing of pills and stuff like that, it would be, just a word of inquiry. . . . The focus seemed to be on how I felt, rather than discharging the responsibility, not "The patient in room 316 is now done," and I can go back to the next chore and so on, it was more to make sure that I really was okay.

Genuine concern for the well-being of the patient includes accepting the patient as he or she is and acknowledging the patient's pain and suffering. The following account illustrates this aspect of caring and also effectively summarizes the patient's perspective on the caring/competence dichotomy:

> Caring experience was mainly where I felt, where the nurse was very competent and knew what she was talking about and doing, and where she didn't deny the fact that you had pain and you were suffering. So there was a level of understanding of what you were going through instead of discarding your feelings and pain, or whatever, discomfort. And the caring part came in, administering of the shots, for example, how that was done was an indication of whether the nurse cared or she didn't care. Coming for a call, the caring ones would always be there sort of in seconds and understand that there was a genuine need, instead of "What the hell do you want now?" kind of thing, which happened as well.

DEVELOPING THE CARING CONCEPT

Margaret J. Dunlop has shaken us out of any conventional thoughts about caring. In 1986, she questioned whether a science of caring is possible. She has taken up the same question again more recently, saying that caring as a concept within nursing is still in the process of being invented or constructed (Dunlop, 1994). She argues that the vast literature on the effects of depersonalization in health, education, and welfare can be seen as a public acknowledgment of the problems of separating "care" from "love," and that the enriched meaning of caring that is emerging can be seen as a way of attempting to solve this problem. She further argues that a central task nursing has taken upon itself is the translation of "love" into the public domain. She warns us, however, that an unexamined adoption of the rhetoric of caring may blind us to its limitations.

I heartily agree that, although it seems possible to claim that nursing is a form of caring, it seems much less reasonable to claim it is *the* form of caring. Such a claim does scant justice to other "people workers," such as teachers, physicians, and physiotherapists (to name only a few), who are endeavoring to overcome the problems caused by the movement of "people work" into the public domain. Dunlop (1994) claims that there is a temptation among nurses to concentrate on either the troubled body or the troubled psyche in order to simplify nursing work. However, what the nursing community means by *good nursing* is neither purely physical nor purely psychosocial. As Dunlop further notes, there is a dematerializing tendency within nursing, a tendency to devalue physical care, as evidenced by the fact that such care has increasingly been delegated to the lower orders of the nursing hierarchy, nurses thus moving toward "cleaner forms of caring." Dunlop criticizes Watson (1979) and other caring theorists for having a tendency to advocate "disembodied caring." She believes that Watson "etherealizes the body" by concentrating her attention on the psychosocial correlates of basic physiological needs, a phenomenon Dunlop (1994) refers to as "logocentric caring" or "a tendency to lose the bedpan" (p. 32).

Dunlop's point is well taken in that an emergent sense of caring that ignores the physical care that nurses provide for their patients is insufficient to provide a framework for guiding nursing practice. However, this critique deserves caution. Despite Watson's (1979, 1985) tendency to emphasize the psychosocial dimension of nursing, I believe that she and other theorists on caring, such as Roach (1987) and Gadow (1985), have done nursing a great favor by making explicit some of the important dimensions of caring, including the moral ideal of protection and enhancement of human dignity, as well as the importance of working from the moral principle of regard for patients as subjects as opposed to objects. The problem, then, lies not in the theories themselves as much as in the overeagerness of many clinical and educational institutions to adopt them as theoretical frameworks encompassing all the dimensions of nursing. Such a framework does not yet exist and perhaps never will. Consequently, theorists can hardly be blamed if their models or theories are inadequate to guide all dimensions of nursing, unless, of course, the theorists themselves claim that they do.

Dunlop (1994) criticizes Watson (1979) and Leininger (1981) for advocating caring in terms of a set of context-free variables. Although her criticism in this respect may not be well grounded, I would agree that comfort, compassion, and concern can never be fully context-free—they are always highly dependent on context. Indeed, we need to listen more carefully to the recipients of nursing care and thereby acquire a deeper understanding of how context influences people's experiences of caring and uncaring encounters with nurses and other health care workers. As Johns (1995) points out, practitioners may have difficulty in applying a knowledge that has been generated within context-free situations and therefore ignores the context of the actual practice situation. Such knowledge must always be interpreted in the context of actual practice. The danger with such knowledge is the notion that it has a universal application and hence can be applied uncritically in all situations (Johns, 1995). Such a viewpoint leads to an image of practice that reduces nurses to technicians who apply rules and procedures to patients in specific situations. In other words, such an image denies the humanness of both the nurse and the patient—"both becoming objects to be manipulated to achieve predicted outcomes" (Johns, 1995, p. 24).

I further believe, as does Dunlop (1994), that caring is profoundly shaped by the social structures of the institutions of care. The way that caring is "cooled out" and subverted in nursing is a real danger to nursing as a caring profession. As Dunlop notes, the qualities that have been nurtured in the traditional world of women should not be lost. I too have a vision of a different sort of society, "perfused by caring," that would be more flexible and attuned to the meeting of human needs. Although, as Dunlop points out, such a society might have a reduced need for nursing, it is a vision that is worth fighting for. However, blaming patients' experiences of uncaring encounters with nurses and other health professionals solely on the system, as Dunlop attempts to do, is an oversimplification of the problem of uncaring. Uncaring in nursing is an ethical as well as a professional problem that nursing has not addressed properly as a profession. The uncomfortable truth is that there are cold people within the caring professions, and even some who are malevolent (Halldórsdóttir, 1996).

A THEORY INVOLVING CARING AND COMPETENCE

As I claimed earlier in this chapter, the urgent need for a science that guides the logic of nursing practice demands the development of proposals for a socially constructed evaluative component to practice science. In an effort to construct this evaluative component, I have been developing a theory based on the nine previously mentioned phenomenological studies (Halldórsdóttir, 1996). My views on the caring/competence dichotomy, as well as my understandings of caring and uncaring, have evolved through my listening to these former recipients of nursing care. From this program of research, I have concluded that competence administered with compassion is an essential component of professional caring from the patient's perspective. I therefore understand caring and compassion to be the underlying forces that make up true professional competence. They are experienced by the patient as genuine concern and capability, and thus there can be no caring/competence dichotomy. In professional caring, competence and caring are inextricably intertwined; deficiencies in either will diminish nursing.

Using the metaphor of a bridge, a caring encounter may be perceived as openness in communication that creates a connection between the professional and the recipient of care. In contrast, the metaphor of a wall serves to illustrate the sense of detachment and lack of connection that can be experienced by the recipient of an uncaring encounter. From the patient's perspective, the essential structure of a caring encounter with a nurse has three basic components: (a) the nurse's professional caring approach; (b) the relationship that develops between the nurse and the patient, which is one of attachment with professional distance (the bridge); and (c) the patient's response to the caring encounter, which can be described as an increased sense of well-being or as healing. The nurse's professional caring approach is a prerequisite of the nurse-patient "bridge building," and together these components form the essential structure of professional caring.

The Nurse's Professional Caring Approach: Competence and Caring

From the perspective of former patients, the nurse's professional caring approach inherently reflects competence and caring, including compassionate competence, genuine concern for the patient, undivided attention when the nurse is with the patient, and an element of openness and responsibility. The caring nurse is skillful, knowledgeable, and committed to the provision of personalized care, and knows how to safeguard the personal integrity and dignity of each person who is a patient. Patients clearly perceive that genuine concern and respect for the individuality and well-being of the patient are important aspects of true professional caring. The manifestations of such attitudes include the nurse's genuinely wishing the patient well, attempting to understand and accept the patient in his or her unique circumstances, acknowledging the patient's pain and suffering, and responding to specific needs.

The essential elements of competence and caring (see Table 7.1) have emerged in our studies as evidence of professional caring. Although it is beyond the scope of this discussion to depict the dark side of human encounters within health care and explain aspects of the theory associated with professional uncaring, as might be predicted, much of that theory reflects the opposite of caring encounters.

Nurse-Patient Attachment With Professional Distance: Building the Bridge

Patient co-researchers in our studies have unanimously perceived that encountering a professionally caring nurse creates in them a sense

TABLE 7.1 Competence and Caring Aspects of Professional Care Within Nursing

The Competence Aspect	*The Caring Aspect*
Competence in empowering people Competence in building relationships Competence in facilitating knowledge development (educating people) Competence in making clinical judgments Competence in doing tasks and taking action on behalf of people (including active advocacy and collaboration)	Being open to life and perceptive of others (being sensitive to patient needs) Being genuinely concerned for the patient, as a person and as a patient Being morally responsible (being respectful of self and others) Being dedicated as a professional nurse Being truly present for the patient (attentiveness to the present moment; being present in a dialogue, in listening and responding; being present in a situation, physically and emotionally)

of trust that facilitates the development of a nurse-patient attachment or relationship. Many former patients considered this connection, or personal relationship, to be the fundamental difference between caring and uncaring.

R: What would you say would be the fundamental difference between caring and uncaring?

C: I'm not sure how to put it other than "personal relationship," the sense is somehow that your and my spirit have met in the experience. And the whole idea that there is somebody in that hospital who is with me, rather than working on me.

Another participant explained it this way:

> You know, there is that kind of bonding, that kind of feeling of . . . not intimacy, but at least connection, there has been a connection made with that person, a connection which I could then follow up on, you know, I would feel free to do so.

Although the professionally caring nurse is both with and for the patient, the nurse maintains separateness throughout the development of attachment. This separateness is what constitutes professional distance, a dimension of professional attachment that has to be present to keep caring in the professional domain. It is apparent from our co-researchers' accounts that this bonding or attachment involves such professional distance. Nurse-patient attachment with professional distance, therefore, involves both of these interrelated processes: developing professional attachment and keeping a professional distance (Halldórsdóttir, 1996).

Keeping a professional distance seems to be an essential aspect of professional caring. As patients, our co-researchers wished not only for professional attachment but also for professional distance. From their point of view, the nurse-patient connection belongs to a particular setting, or culture, and should be confined to that setting. Furthermore, they have emphasized that keeping a professional distance is one important way of keeping the nurse-patient connection within the professional domain.

Patient Responses to Professional Caring

It is evident from our data that patients' reactions to professional caring are very positive. The outcome of professional caring is positive change—an increased sense of well-being and health. The professional nurse gets to know the patient as a unique individual and treats the patient accordingly, communicating with the patient in a way that makes the patient feel accepted as a normal human being and legitimated as a person and as a patient. This helps the patient to feel all right about him- or herself and the health care encounter. One former patient described it in the following way:

> I think it's very important that you emotionally and mentally yourself be . . . accentuating the health in you, you know, not being dragged down mentally and emotionally by your disease, and that whatever happens to you, ahh . . . becomes all right, let's use the word legiti-

> mized. If you shit your pants, you know, somehow that's got to be legitimized so that's not something that says to you, "Oh, God, look who I am now, look what's happened to me now," you know. "Now I'm just one step further down the ladder," you know. And a nurse can do that for you, she can help to legitimize it. . . . There was [a] nurse who really did that for me, when that happened, you know. Just her, her attitude just seemed, "Oh, sure, okay." It wasn't breezy, it wasn't, she wasn't absent from the situation, but she somehow just made it all okay, it was okay and she understood my upset, she didn't brush that away, but she did still in some way give me the message that "you don't have to be that upset," you know. So, that caring is very important to help me work on my own health.

Professional caring seems to give the patient a sense of hope and optimism, encouragement, and reassurance. It results in relaxation and gives the patient a sense of security. Professional caring decreases the patient's anxiety, increases the patient's confidence, and positively affects the patient's sense of well-being and healing. The accounts of our co-researchers further suggest that caring may even represent a matter of life or death for the patient; that is, when the patient does not get any encouragement he or she may in fact lose the will to live. One former patient explained this in the following way:

> I guess my feeling was, just some relief that I was being cared for. But I think in the absence of it I would have felt very alone and very depressed, and could well have gotten sick because of that, or gotten sicker. In fact, it strikes me that it wouldn't take much depression before I became indifferent to whether or not I recovered, and that could easily become a self-fulfilling prophecy, I mean if I didn't have the will to live, I mean the likelihood that drugs would force me to live might be remote, because I was very sick, and without the will, who knows?

As is evident from their accounts, our participants were very grateful for the professional caring they received. Because of such caring, they carried pleasant memories away from their hospital stays, sometimes the only pleasant memories they had of their hospitalizations (Halldórsdóttir, 1996).

PROFESSIONAL CARING

Recipients of nursing seek professional nurses because of their professional expertise. If we ignore competence as an essential element in our professional caring, we undermine the expertise patients require (Bishop & Scudder, 1996). However, instead of "mass-production-line processing" and "emotional sterility" (Lowenberg, 1994), true competence requires professional caring. In articulating problems associated with a caring/competence dichotomy, nursing is well placed to demonstrate leadership among health care professions in explicating the complexities inherent in provider-recipient relationships that facilitate outcomes such as healing and health.

The studies discussed in this chapter underscore the need for a shift toward a more egalitarian, less hierarchical stance between nurses and the recipients of nursing care, to give the recipients of care authority and control within the interaction, in what Lowenberg (1994) describes as "a model of partnership." In contrast to the parent-child tradition (described by Sidenvall, 1995), such interactions must proceed reciprocally, as between two adults of comparable status. Whereas nurses have often deplored the "paternalistic" tendencies of their physician colleagues, they ignore their own "maternalistic" tendencies toward using power differentials to control patients. As Lowenberg points out, our professional discourse, including the use of such terms as *allow* and *compliance,* reveals evidence of such tendencies.

According to Meleis (1992), the development of the discipline of nursing has gone through four stages: theorizing, syntax development, concept development, and philosophical debate. These stages have shaped the characteristics of the discipline as a human science, a practice science, and a science with social goals to empower nurses, to empower the discipline, and to empower the recipients of nursing care. The ideas presented in this chapter could provide a basis for improving these practical and social goals by alerting us to the concerns of health care recipients that might not be captured through other forms of evaluation. As Johns (1995) contends, it is only through reflection on experience that the practitioner can meaningfully assimilate research findings into practice and that "the 'personal,' the 'ethical,' and the 'aesthetic' ways of knowing can be known and developed" (p. 25). I hope that the conclusions I have drawn from my studies can aid such reflection.

To close this chapter, one former patient's comments about a caring nurse capture the essence of what professional caring entails:

> I expect her to have a basic knowledge of what she's doing, that she empathizes with me, and knows what's going on inside me, at least physically, and hopefully mentally. That she is accepting of all the emotions and also the physical things that are happening. That she shows caring toward me and also toward my family. . . . Respect for me as a human being, and . . . I like a sense of humor.

The way we see our world is modified by our philosophy, as a pair of glasses modifies our vision. The emerging theory of professional caring within nursing can serve as a tentative analytic framework amenable to ongoing reconstruction in the light of new data and changes in nursing philosophy. As our worldview evolves, a theory such as this will always be in a process of emergence. Although our modern technological world appears to confront us with an unavoidable trade-off between competence and caring, a progressive view of professional nursing that includes both competence and caring is required to guide nursing's art and science. Nursing must come to terms with the knowledge that, as it has the power to empower, it also has the power to cause harm. Professional caring permits nurses to enter into the patient's healing process and thereby to manifest its social mandate toward an increased level of health.

REFERENCES

Bishop, A. H., & Scudder, J. R., Jr. (1996). *Nursing ethics: Therapeutic caring presence.* Sudbury, MA: Jones & Bartlett.

Bottorff, J. L. (1991). Nursing: A practical science of caring. *Advances in Nursing Science, 14*(1), 26-39.

Clifford, C. (1995). Caring: Fitting the concept to nursing practice. *Journal of Clinical Nursing, 4,* 37-41.

Dunlop, M. J. (1986). Is a science of caring possible? *Journal of Advanced Nursing, 11,* 661-670.

Dunlop, M. J. (1994). Is a science of caring possible? In P. Benner (Ed.), *Interpretive phenomenology: Embodiment, caring, and ethics in health and illness.* Thousand Oaks, CA: Sage.

Gadow, S. (1985). Nurse and patient: The caring relationship. In A. H. Bishop & J. R. Scudder, Jr. (Eds.), *Caring, curing, coping: Nurse, physician, patient relationships.* University: University of Alabama Press.

Gutierrez-Calleros, G. (1992). The secret of caring in medicine. *Humane Medicine, 8,* 148-151.

Halldórsdóttir, S. (1988). *The essential structure of a caring and an uncaring encounter with a nurse: From the client's perspective.* Unpublished master's thesis, University of British Columbia, Vancouver.

Halldórsdóttir, S. (1990). The essential structure of a caring and an uncaring encounter with a nurse: The patient's perspective. In B. Schultz (Ed.), *Nursing research for professional practice* (pp. 308-333). Frankfurt: German Nursing Association.

Halldórsdóttir, S. (1996). *Caring and uncaring encounters in nursing and health care: Developing a theory.* Unpublished doctoral dissertation, Linköping University, Sweden, Department of Caring Sciences.

Hawthorne, D. L., & Yurkovich, N. J. (1995). Science, technology, caring and the professions: Are they compatible? *Journal of Advanced Nursing, 21,* 1087-1091.

Jarrett, N., & Payne, S. (1995). A selective review of the literature on nurse-patient communication: Has the patient's contribution been neglected? *Journal of Advanced Nursing, 22,* 72-78.

Johns, C. (1995). The value of reflective practice for nursing. *Journal of Clinical Nursing, 4,* 23-30.

Jones, C. B., & Alexander, J. W. (1993). The technology of caring: A synthesis of technology and caring for nursing administration. *Nursing Administration Quarterly, 17*(2), 11-20.

Käppeli, S. (1993). Advanced clinical practice: How do we promote it? *Journal of Advanced Nursing, 20,* 205-210.

Koch, R. (1994). Beyond measurement: Fourth-generation evaluation in nursing. *Journal of Advanced Nursing, 20,* 1148-1155.

Leininger, M. M. (1981). The phenomenon of caring: Importance, research questions and theoretical considerations. In M. M. Leininger (Ed.), *Caring: An essential human need.* Thorofare, NJ: Charles B. Slack.

Locsin, R. C. (1995). Machine technologies and caring in nursing. *Image: The Journal of Nursing Scholarship, 27,* 201-203.

Lowenberg, J. S. (1994). The nurse-patient relationship reconsidered: An expanded research agenda. *Scholarly Inquiry for Nursing Practice, 8,* 167-184.

Meleis, A. I., (1992). Directions for nursing theory development in the 21st century. *Nursing Science Quarterly, 5,* 112-117.

Morse, J. M., Bottorff, J., Neander, W., & Solberg, S. (1991). Comparative analysis of conceptualizations and theories of caring. *Image: The Journal of Nursing Scholarship, 23,* 119-126.

Oldroyd, D. (1989). *The arch of knowledge: An introductory study of the history of the philosophy and methodology of science.* Kensington: New South Wales University Press.

Rawnsley, M. M. (1994). Response to "The nurse-patient relationship reconsidered: An expanded research agenda." *Scholarly Inquiry for Nursing Practice, 8,* 184-190.

Roach, S. (1987). *The human act of caring: A blueprint for the health professions.* Ottawa: Canadian Hospital Association.

Sidenvall, B. (1995). *The meal in geriatric care: Habits, values and culture.* Unpublished doctoral dissertation, Linköping University, Sweden, Department of Caring Sciences.

Watson, J. (1979). *Nursing: The philosophy and science of caring.* Boston: Little, Brown.

Watson, J. (1985). *Nursing: Human science and human care.* Norwalk, CT: Appleton-Century-Crofts.

Thinking Nursing

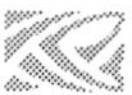

MARION JONES

This chapter explores the assumptions and beliefs underlying the theory-practice gap debate. These assumptions and beliefs are derived from the literature, knowledge development itself, the ongoing struggle for professional identity, and the interrelationships among these. The theory-practice gap is a recurring theme in the literature. It is seen as the distancing of theoretical knowledge from the actual doing of practice. A polarization between theory and practice is generally accepted, and there are many schools of thought as to how they may be integrated and reconciled (Cook, 1991; McCaugherty, 1991; Miller, 1985). One factor contributing to this polarization is an antitheoretical bias that has existed since the early 1960s. Although this bias is less obvious today than it was in the past, it persists and is evident in the lack of understanding of such terms as *theory, concept, model,* and *framework.* It is evident that the theory-practice gap debate is not an issue for nursing alone, as other disciplines, such as education and psychology, are wrestling with similar issues (Speedy, 1989b). McCaugherty (1991) argues that the theory-practice gap in nursing has never been accurately described, and many unanswered questions remain.

Nursing uses many types of knowledge to achieve its goals. Meleis (1991) sees the purposes of knowledge development as "empowerment of the discipline of nursing; empowerment of the nurses; and empowerment of clients to care for themselves to take advantage of the resources available to them" (p. 129). If nursing is to progress in this way, nurses need to examine further the forces that have shaped their professional practice. According to the nursing literature, these forces include the struggles for accountability, autonomy, recognition of responsibility, and control over the development of the profession (Bent, 1993; Kozier, Erb, & Blais, 1992; Miller, 1985; Strasen, 1992). It is possible that such practice problems could be resolved if nurses begin to "think nursing."

"Thinking nursing" involves the interweaving of the skills, values, norms, and nursing knowledge that provide the basis for development of the profession (Perry, 1985). Perry (1985) asks which skills, which beliefs and attitudes, and what kind of knowledge allow the nurse to think nursing. The options are influenced by the way an individual views the world in relation to knowledge development and clinical practice. Influences on a nurse's thinking nursing include professional socialization; the social, cultural, and political stances taken by the nurse; and the nurse's perceived worldview, which guides his or her practice. As the knowledge base of the nurse increases, nursing identity strengthens and the place of cognitive, behavioral, and affective skills becomes interrelated and interdependent. Therefore, a component of thinking nursing is an interdependence of skills, knowledge, attitudes, values, and professional identity that allows complex thinking to occur. Perry considers such thinking the most complex form of human behavior, because it is reliant upon physiological coordination of neural responses as well as cognitive processes characterized by the use of symbols as representations of objects and events.

Nursing practice encompasses clinical practice, theory/knowledge development, and educational practice (Jones, 1993). Praxis is theory and practice that are interrelated, integrated, and dialectal in nature. Inherent within praxis is reflection both on and in practice. Reflection has the potential to enhance self-awareness and increase the possibility for change. Carr and Kemmis (1986) assert that praxis is informed action, simultaneously the action and the knowledge that informs it. In the dynamic environment of change and complexity in clinical practice, thought and action are intrinsically linked and mutually dependent. Praxis includes deliberate action by which a theory or philosophy becomes integrated into the social reality of the practice environment (Bawden, 1989). Nurses have the power to determine the directions they wish to take in this dynamic environment; they can maintain the status quo or choose liberation, emancipation, and freedom to practice within an environment characterized by adaptation, flexibility, and a horizontal power that does not perpetuate the perceived powerlessness of nurses (Hall, Stevens, & Meleis, 1994; Henderson, 1995; Jones, 1993; Roberts, 1983).

NURSING'S HISTORY OF THEORY AND KNOWLEDGE DEVELOPMENT

Florence Nightingale first identified nursing as an art and a science, believing that both were equally important (Cull-Wilby & Pepin, 1987). Nightingale not only began the development of nursing as a discipline, but also stressed the importance of nursing education. For the rest of the nineteenth century and into the twentieth, one main theoretical model evolved—logical empiricism. The medical model, derived from logical empiricism, in turn encompassed societal beliefs from a time when women were subordinate to men. Such a patriarchal view is still evident in the health professions today. With logical empiricists valuing the results of scientific inquiry more than the process of the science, the nursing theories developed were aimed at describing, explaining, and predicting phenomena as well as at showing relationships between them (Carr & Kemmis, 1986; Chinn & Jacobs, 1983). The early 1950s witnessed a boom in nursing theories, expanding the body of nursing knowledge on the basis of logical positivism and borrowed theory from other disciplines. "Nursing partly lost sight of the importance of the art of nursing and concentrated primarily on the science of nursing" (Cull-Wilby & Pepin, 1987, p. 517).

By the 1980s, the logical empiricist approach was being challenged within nursing circles. The transfer of nursing education from hospital-based apprentice style to preparation of students within an educational institution was well established in some parts of the world. Systems theory and humanistic perspectives had become theoretical alternatives that held the development of each individual's unique potential and issues of personal, cultural, and societal well-being paramount. Ideological perspectives broadened to include socioeconomic-political approaches and later feminist and critical social theory approaches. Many nurses expressed a sense of disquiet about the way in which the practice of nursing reflected an unbalanced emphasis on the biomedical model and technological concerns, neglecting concern for the lived experiences of clients.

Critical social theory is an approach that involves sociopolitical critique and has the aim of transforming society rather than maintaining the status quo. The advantage of critical science for nursing is that it offers an opportunity to shatter the ideological mirror that traps nurses and their clients in despair and hopelessness. "Taken seriously, it forces us to question that status quo at every turn, sifting and winnowing our personal and working lives to enable us to formulate a truly alternative plan" (Allen, 1985, p. 64). Similarly, a feminist approach recognizes everyday experiences as "inextricably connected to the larger political, social and economic environment" (Hall & Stevens, 1991, p. 18). Although these approaches reflect alternative views of theory and practice (Carr & Kemmis, 1986), it has been argued that their uncritical application could seriously impede the creativity and autonomy needed to promote professional practice in a changing environment. For example, although these new paradigms have driven curriculum and research development, attempts to introduce them into practice may create a double bind (Carr & Kemmis, 1986; Watson, 1981). In keeping with the tradition of nursing theory development, the apparent gap between theory and practice can therefore be wide, variant, polarizing, and confusing. However, a focus on the dichotomy between theory and practice is counterproductive when its basis is not understood. Further, in maintaining the view of a theory-practice gap, we may endorse and maintain the structures of a positivist paradigm (Street, 1990).

WAYS OF KNOWING AND KNOWLEDGE DEVELOPMENT

Nursing is a complex and varied discipline, and no single theory is able to answer all the questions of practice. Many theories have evolved that encompass both the shared meanings and diverse views of nursing. Nursing has developed a knowledge base that emphasizes the structure of knowledge more than its content (Meleis, 1992). Carper (1978) identifies four patterns of knowing: empirics, the science of nursing; aesthetics, the art of nursing; the component of personal knowledge of nursing; and ethics, the component of moral knowledge in nursing. These ways of knowing are interdependent and interrelated, reflecting the diversity of knowledge and the ever-changing dynamic knowledge base of nursing practice in the 1990s. Within practice settings, nurses are still coming to terms with the complexity of nursing and its ability to take its rightful place as an evolving discipline. Cull-Wilby and Pepin (1987) contend that, although nursing is a profession of nurturing and human interaction within a social context, its scholars have retained traditional and inappropriate methods for exploring, explaining, and predicting phenomena. Thus it is essential to reflect on the epistemology of nursing knowledge in order to gain a clearer view of our theoretical progress to date and the future development directions that can be predicted (Meleis, 1991).

THEORY AND PRACTICE: WHAT ARE THEY?

Ways of knowing and theory development have become large issues with which nurses should become familiar and then use as a base for their practice. The desired effects are that theory will influence practice and that nursing practice will contribute to theory development (Sparacino, 1991). The term *theory* can be interpreted in many ways. The tendency to perceive theory as different from practice represents a dichotomy between *what is* and *what ought to be done.* Typically, theories are aimed at explaining, predicting, and organizing knowledge about nursing practice (Chinn & Jacobs, 1983; Stevens-

Barnum, 1990). Other interpretations of the distinction between theory and practice include the differentiation between theoretical and practical nursing; for example, nursing's scholarly writing is sometimes judged as being "too theoretical," betraying an anti-intellectual focus within practice. In this case, theory is seen as knowledge, whereas practice is action. From such a perspective, theory can be seen as distinct from practice and as involving activities that are separate. Alternatively, theory can be seen as the principles that underlie practice, demonstrating that theory and practice are interrelated to make a unified nursing discipline. In this manner, theory may evolve from practice as practice may evolve from theory (Stevens-Barnum, 1990), and theory and practice depend upon each other for development (Moccia, 1992). Theory can be seen as informing and transforming practice by informing and transforming the ways in which practice is experienced and understood. "The transition is not, therefore, from theory to practice as such, but rather from irrationality to rationality, from ignorance and habit to knowledge and reflection" (Carr & Kemmis, 1986, p. 116). Using this perspective, nursing theory is a way of describing and explaining what nursing is, like a road map that provides perspective or guidance for action (Stevens, 1989). According to Meleis (1991), "Theory is an organized, coherent, and systematic articulation of a set of statements related to significant questions in a discipline that are communicated in a meaningful whole" (p. 12). Similarly, many definitions within the literature focus on nursing theory from a perspective of structure, practice goal, research, or nursing phenomena, offering frameworks for practice.

On the other hand, practice is seen as the action, knowing "how to," and the reality of nursing as it is (Miller, 1985). Practice displays the action that theory affirms in words, and together "the theoretical affirmation and the effective practice develop dialectically at any one time in what Gramsci (1971) calls an 'ensemble of relations' " (Moccia, 1992, p. 35). Whereas some see practice as the source of theory, others believe that theory guides practice (Speedy, 1989b). From a positivist philosophy, however, practice can be seen as technical when the doing and the deciding are kept separate (Schön, 1992). With this variance in the understanding of theory and practice, it is not surprising to find an asserted dichotomy between theory and practice still used as a rationale for maintaining the status quo and the power imbalances often evidenced within bureaucratic organizational structures.

CULTURE OF NURSING

In exploring the theory-practice debate within nursing, it becomes apparent that some issues related to the historical trends of theory development and the place of women in professions should be considered within the context of nursing culture. Culture may be defined as a "set of definitions of reality held in common by a group of individuals who share a distinctive way of life" (Strasen, 1992, p. 3). Ideology, personal knowledge, power, and professional judgment are influenced by the culture of nursing. Within culture are the crucial elements of shared values, beliefs, expectations, attitudes, assumptions, and norms. Often these are not written about, discussed, or recognized, as they are lived and internalized as norms that provide social signposts for behavior. Nursing culture includes the practices, beliefs, knowledge, language, and resources that are particular to nursing, in addition to its involvement in hierarchical power relationships with medical culture, allied health professionals, and educationalists (Lovell, 1980; Sohier, 1992; Street, 1992). As in the evolution of nursing as a practice discipline it was generally accepted that women were subordinate to men, nurses were seen in the role of ministering to and caring for everyone within a hospital, including doctors as well as patients (Buckingham & McGrath, 1983). For nurses joining a new unit, practice, or institution, their socialization into their responsibilities became an issue of acculturation.

Within the shared cultural dimensions of nursing practice, specialized language or jargon is often a predominant identifying feature. To illustrate, nurses new to a specific practice setting often feel isolated, devalued, and ineffective until they master the specialized language of that unit. In order to unravel what lies behind or within language, nurses need to question the motives, values, desires, and assumptions underlying it. As a social construction, language can be a subtle and powerful tool for controlling behavior. For example, control through the use of language has been shown to have the effect of disempowering nurses and re-creating the hegemony of medical dominance (Street, 1992). The use of specialized language can also perpetuate the theory-practice gap by signaling distinctions between theorists and practitioners through the use of such jargon terms as *self-care agents, energy fields,* and *paradigms of thinking* (Meleis, 1991; Street, 1992). When we begin to understand the effects of language, we can start to foster acceptance and peer support (Jones, 1993). The challenge for nurses is to apply this appreciation toward the broader issue of empowering each other.

Research indicates that women tend toward low self-esteem and self-image, which directly influences performance, motivation, and relationships (Strasen 1992). The struggle for nursing to separate from the medical profession and to see the roles of the nurses and physicians as complementary has been magnified by male domination of the medical profession (Strasen, 1992). As a result, nurses still see themselves as being socialized for dependence on others and avoid challenging the power of bureaucracy and hierarchy. Street (1992) argues that the single most important factor maintaining the oppression that nurses experience continues to be the reification of Florence Nightingale's nursing regime of hierarchy, compliance, and obedience. Viewing nurses as an oppressed group, Roberts (1983) suggests that nurses reject or hide their own culture as a means of dealing with their negative feelings about it. This may explain why the internalized values of medicine have been evidenced in the development of nursing theory and in its use of medical model concepts that reinforce the dominance of a positivist paradigm.

Power and knowledge are interrelated, and where leadership is strong, knowledge continues to develop. Thus knowledge, language, and self-esteem are important components of social power. For example, pressure from management within health care for evidence of a theory base to show how nursing makes a difference has bulldozed some nurses into using frameworks that they do not fully understand or feel committed to, that they feel do not reflect the humanistic values of nursing, or that they believe are restrictive to practice. It has also been suggested that a significant element of nursing culture that furthers nurses' disempowerment is their adherence to a culture that favors oral transmission of practices over written transmission in the belief that oral communication saves time. Perry (1987) claims that nurses' reluctance to document their knowledge and skills in writing has resulted in limitations to their access to channels of power. Discomfort with written language therefore immobilizes nurses in their knowledge development and critique and perpetuates the traditional myths and rituals that maintain the status quo.

THEORY-PRACTICE DEBATE

The literature portrays nurses as perceiving the theory-practice gap as an important issue for research and as seeking its resolution for the very survival of nursing as we know it today (Benner, 1984; Meleis, 1991; Miller, 1985; Stevens-Barnum, 1990). The stance I take is that nurses must change the thinking that perpetuates their seeing practice as the "doing" at the bedside and theory as a separate entity. Nurse educators are often criticized as being full of the jargon of academia, whereas nurse clinicians are seen as using more reality-based language. Miller (1985) notes that these "two groups of nurses have different perceptions of patients and of nursing and do value different kinds of nursing knowledge" (p. 417). As Meleis (1991) has observed, "In the minds of practitioners, theorists who were associated with the ivory towers of educational institutions were castigated for being far removed from practice" (p. 43). Using the language of difference between theory and practice, nurses may excuse their failures to change how they work or think. However, in resisting change, nurses decrease their own autonomy and may ignore their self-responsibility for upgrading or extending knowledge. They allow a hegemonic situation to exist because they do not perceive what they do and how they "practice nursing" as needing change. The context in which nurses practice and the ways in which society changes cannot be ignored. However difficult change may be for nurses, they must acknowledge and accommodate it by being flexible and adaptable, changing their ways of thinking about clinical nursing practice, and developing new knowledge.

Because nurses reproduce the culture of nursing when they interact with others in multiple settings and in different ways, an apparent theory-practice debate may not be a matter of knowledge or skill, but may be one of expectations. In Smyth's (1986) view, "By continuing to insist on using such phrases as the translation of theory into practice, closing the gap between theory and practice, and integrating theory and practice, we are still fundamentally wedded to the idea that theory and practice are separate" (p. 11). A change in the way that nurses think nursing and a recognition of the cultural context in which nursing occurs may influence the interpretations and assumptions of the actual day-to-day practice of nursing. Jones (1993) suggests that nurses need to examine the power of the myths and rituals of present-day nursing in light of their historical context.

Schön (1983) believes that, through reflection in action, professionals make sense of value conflicts, current practice uncertainties, and the uniqueness of self and colleagues. Traditionally, nurses have been socialized toward self-images that value giving, caring, and dedication (Strasen, 1992). Today's dominant hierarchical social structures of health and education reflect a technical positivist ideology that is evidenced in control, competition, profit, efficiency, and effectiveness. These features are not conducive to the reflection, challenge, and critical analysis that are encouraged for today's nurses. Until nurses explicitly acknowledge the process of knowledge development, especially in relation to professional self-esteem and nursing culture, it would appear that "gap" language and ideal/reality debates will persist.

WAYS OF THINKING THEORY-PRACTICE

Theory-practice issues related to professional judgment can be interpreted as the professional work of the nurse and therefore the totality of nursing in whatever setting. The coexistence of different paradigms of thinking affects the assumptions and judgments of nurses, including how and what nurses perceive as being theory-practice and whether or not a gap exists (Cull-Wilby & Pepin, 1987). Emphasizing a gap creates the impression that praxis is not valued. Thus, as long as the idea of the "gap" is evident in our day-to-day practice language, the separation of theory and practice is perpetuated.

Moccia (1992) asserts that nursing theorists would do better to account for a dialectical relationship instead of perpetuating endless papers and conferences in which a gap between education and clinical service is depicted. Nursing needs to delete the word *gap* from its lexicon and use an interactive model in which practice is seen as a developmental process incorporating praxis for growth (Jones, 1993). Within this view, it would be acknowledged that each nursing practice grouping develops its own unique culture of shared beliefs, values, myths, knowledge, and processes of doing. Along with providing the affective, cognitive, and behavioral skills of nursing knowledge, this unique culture helps give the nurse the capacity to "think nursing." Perry (1985) believes that nurses already think nursing, "but from a variety of conceptual orientations—medical, physical and technological—which incorporate some nursing concepts. Differences between theoretical approaches should be seen for what they are, that is, a commitment to a particular way of 'thinking nursing' based on social, political and ideological positions" (p. 37).

Acknowledging nursing practice as a developmental process is a means of valuing the expertise of all nurses at all levels between novice and expert (Benner, 1984). Speedy (1989a) emphasizes that the derivation of theory from practice and its reciprocal nature are vital for developing multiple ways of understanding our world. As Chinn (1989) notes, "Whether we call it practice oriented theory, or putting an idea into practice—we are describing praxis" (p. 74). By acknowledging praxis as an integral process within nursing practice, we can transform nursing thinking.

Theory is not an end in itself; the belief that it is perpetuates a gap and promotes the distinction between theory and practice. This separation causes theory to be seen as esoteric and fragments nursing educational and clinical practice. Chinn (1989) asserts that if nurses are ever going to be able to achieve unity between their knowing and doing, they must increase their conviction that this can be achieved and begin to take responsibility to heal the theory-practice split. If thinking nursing becomes an ideal goal of nursing practice, the dichotomy of theory and practice no longer exists.

A number of strategies could facilitate the change in thinking needed for this dynamic model of empowerment for nurses. These include ongoing education, collaborative education programs between education and service, coaching and clinical supervision, mentoring, reflection, case management, faculty practice, research, and reciprocal advisory groups for both clinical practice and education settings. It is beyond the scope of this chapter for me to elaborate on these strategies individually, but a body of literature exists in relation to each.

Speedy (1989a, 1989b) recognizes the importance of ongoing education for the promotion of the concept of reflection in practice and therefore professional development and the ability to think nursing. As part of changing ways of thinking, reflection on practice can help nurses to recognize imbalances in power relationships and nursing's domination by other groups (Speedy, 1989a). Acknowledgment that there are different ways of knowing (Belenky, Clinchy, Goldberger, & Tarule, 1986; Carper, 1978) can help to legitimate and justify the technique of reflecting on practice, which is essential for understanding and analyzing the theory that is embedded within it (Speedy, 1989b). Critical reflection helps the thinker to discover the historical, traditional, and ideological ways of changing and misinterpreting knowledge and action, along with how these affect the processes of practice. Nurses need to ask themselves whose interests are being served, and how the present situation is affected.

Collaboration between service (clinical practice) and education promotes interdependence between the two practice areas and helps to decrease the theory-practice gap, encouraging nurses to begin to think nursing. Coaching and clinical supervision are indispensable in helping nurses to think nursing, through collaborative planning to identify needs, implementation of plans into action, analysis of the process, reflection on the analysis, and replanning of future strategies. In helping to integrate theory and practice it seems important to use mentoring strategies, which may also help facilitate role development in the realities of the work setting and the political scene (Cooper, 1990; Hagerty, 1986; Playko, 1991). In advancing the discipline of nursing through praxis and thinking nursing, faculty practice and case management can improve outcomes for clients, help consolidate nursing practice, and promote collaborative practice.

CONCLUSION

In deleting the word *gap* from nursing language, theory-practice becomes theory practice, or praxis, demonstrating that theory and practice share a co-determining interaction that promotes professional growth, development, and change through dialogue. Nurses need to ask questions that promote emancipatory nursing action and praxis: Who maintains a particular situation? Who does our current practice serve? How does our nursing culture influence our understanding of the situation? Does progress require that we relinquish comfort and confidence? How do we come to believe in what we do and think? And how do we create partnerships with other nurses, other disciplines, our patients, and our society? In order to understand the world of nursing and the processes involved in thinking nursing, all nurses need to value theory *and* practice. A praxis orientation can be an important step toward our collective ability to think nursing.

REFERENCES

Allen, D. G. (1985). Nursing research and social control: Alternative models of science that emphasize understanding and emancipation. *Image: The Journal of Nursing Scholarship, 17,* 58-64.

Bawden, R. (1989). Praxis: The essence of systems for being. In A. R. Viskovic (Ed.), *Research and development in higher education* (pp. 1-7). Campbelltown, NSW: Herdsa.

Belenky, M. F., Clinchy, B. M., Goldberger, N. R., & Tarule, J. M. (1986). *Women's ways of knowing: The development of self, voice, and mind.* New York: Basic Books.

Benner, P. (1984). *From novice to expert: Excellence and power in clinical nursing practice.* Menlo Park, CA: Addison-Wesley.

Bent, K. N. (1993). Perspectives on critical and feminist theory in developing nursing praxis. *Journal of Professional Nursing, 9,* 296-303.

Buckingham, J. E., & McGrath, G. (1983). *The social reality of nursing.* Balgowlah, NSW: Adis Health Science.

Carper, B. A. (1978). Fundamental patterns of knowing. *Advances in Nursing Science, 1*(1), 13-23.

Carr, W., & Kemmis, S. (1986). *Becoming critical: Knowing through action research.* Geelong, Victoria, Australia: Deakin University Press.

Chinn, P. L. (1989). Nursing patterns of knowing and feminist thought. *Nursing and Health Care, 10,* 71-75.

Chinn, P. L., & Jacobs, M. (1983). *Theory and nursing: A systematic approach.* St. Louis, MO: C. V. Mosby.

Cook, S. H. (1991). Mind the theory/practice gap in nursing. *Journal of Advanced Nursing, 16,* 1462-1469.

Cooper, M. D. (1990). Mentorship: The key to the future of professionalism in nursing. *Journal of Perinatal and Neonatal Nursing, 4*(3), 71-77.

Cull-Wilby, B. L., & Pepin, J. C. (1987). Towards a co-existence of paradigms in nursing knowledge development. *Journal of Advanced Nursing, 12,* 515-521.

Hagerty, B. (1986). A second look at mentors. *Nursing Outlook, 34,* 16-19.

Hall, J. M., & Stevens, P. E. (1991). Rigor in feminist research. *Advances in Nursing Science, 13*(3), 16-29.

Hall, J. M., Stevens, P. E., & Meleis, A. I. (1994). Marginalization: A guiding concept for valuing diversity in nursing knowledge development. *Advances in Nursing Science, 16*(4), 23-41.

Henderson, D. J. (1995). Consciousness raising in participatory research: Method and methodology for emancipatory nursing inquiry. *Advances in Nursing Science, 17*(3), 58-69.

Jones, E. M. (1993). *Shaping nursing praxis: Some registered nurses' perceptions and beliefs of theory practice.* Unpublished master's thesis, Massey University, Palmerston North, New Zealand.

Kozier, B., Erb, A., & Blais, K. (1992). *Concepts and issues in nursing* (2nd ed.). Menlo Park, CA: Addison-Wesley.

Lovell, M. C. (1980). The politics of medical deception: Challenging the trajectory of history. *Advances in Nursing Science, 2*(3), 73-86.

McCaugherty, D. (1991). The theory-practice gap in nurse education: Its course and possible solutions. *Journal of Advanced Nursing, 16,* 1055-1061.

Meleis, A. I. (1991). *Theoretical nursing: Development and progress.* Philadelphia: J. B. Lippincott.

Meleis, A. I. (1992). Theory development and domain concepts in approaches to theory development. In P. Moccia (Ed.), *New approaches to theory development* (pp. 3-21). New York: National League for Nursing.

Miller, A. (1985). The relationship between nursing theory and nursing practice. *Journal of Advanced Nursing, 10,* 417-424.

Moccia, P. (1992). Theory development and nursing practice: A synopsis of a study of the theory-practice dialectic. In P. Moccia (Ed.), *New approaches to theory development* (pp. 23-38). New York: National League for Nursing.

Perry, J. (1985). Has the discipline of nursing developed to the stage where nurses do "think nursing"? *Journal of Advanced Nursing, 10,* 31-37.

Perry, J. (1987). Creating our own image. *New Zealand Nursing Journal, 80*(2), 10-13.

Playko, M. A. (1991). Mentors for administrators: Support for the instructional leader. *Theory into Practice, 30,* 124-127.

Roberts, S. J. (1983). Oppressed group behavior: Implications for nursing. *Advances in Nursing Science, 5*(4), 21-30.

Schön, D. (1983). *The reflective practitioner.* New York: Basic Books.

Schön, D. (1992). The crisis of professional knowledge and the pursuit of an epistemology of practice. *Journal of Interprofessional Care, 6*(1), 49-63.

Smyth, J. (1986). *The reflective practitioner in nurse education.* Unpublished manuscript, Deakin University, Geelong, Victoria, Australia.

Sohier, R. (1992). Feminism and nursing knowledge: The power of the weak. *Nursing Outlook, 40,* 62-66.

Sparacino, P. (1991). The reciprocal relationship between practice and theory. *Clinical Nurse Specialist, 5*(3), 138.

Speedy, S. (1989a). *Monograph of theory and practice: An evolving relationship.* Adelaide: South Australian College of Advanced Education, School of Nursing Studies.

Speedy, S. (1989b). Theory-practice debate: Setting the scene. *Australian Journal of Advanced Nursing, 6*(3), 12-20.

Stevens, P. E. (1989). A critical social reconceptualization of environment in nursing: Implications for methodology. *Advances in Nursing Science, 11*(4), 56-68.

Stevens-Barnum, B. J. (1990). *Nursing theory: Analysis, application, evaluation* (3rd ed.). Glenview, IL: Scott, Foresman/Little, Brown.

Strasen, L. (1992). *The image of professional nursing.* Philadelphia: J. B. Lippincott.

Street, A. (1990). *Nursing practice: High, hard ground, messy swamps and the pathways in between.* Geelong, Victoria, Australia: Deakin University Press.

Street, A. (1992). *Cultural practices in nursing.* Geelong, Victoria, Australia: Deakin University Press.

Watson, J. (1981). Nursing's scientific quest. *Nursing Outlook, 29,* 413-416.

9

Multiple Paradigms for Nursing

Postmodern Feminisms

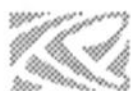

SUELLEN MILLER

Over the past two decades, nursing scholars have called for a greater multiplicity of paradigms, methods and theories that can adequately reflect the complexity of the discipline. The necessity for this multiplicity has become even more acute as we grapple with the increasing complexity of individuals' and communities' lives and health. Watson (1995) has observed that postmodern perspectives, which reflect our fragmented, complex lives and a multiplicity of realities rather than the notion of one truth, are appropriate perspectives for nursing knowledge development. However, nursing researchers, theorists, and philosophers have been slow to adopt postmodern perspectives (Dzurec, 1989; Lister, 1991).

Feminisms have long been accepted among the many schools of thought influencing nursing research and practice (Bunting & Campbell, 1990). Although theorists and researchers in other disciplines are combining feminisms and postmodernisms to gain the complexity of these multiple perspectives, few in nursing have written about combining them (Anderson, 1991; Dickson, 1990; Doering, 1992; Miller, 1994). Yet postmodern feminist perspectives can add layers of complexity and multiplicity to modes of nursing research, methodologies, and epistemologies. In particular, these perspectives provide nurse scientists with the ability to go beyond empiricism and historicism (Thompson, 1985), objectivism and relativism (Bernstein, 1983), and logical positivism and phenomenology/hermeneutics (Dzurec, 1989) and into more contemporary debates within the academy.

Critically combining the perspectives of feminism and postmodernism could enrich nursing knowledge and praxis. To do so, the nursing scientist must understand basic postmodern concepts (often worded in convoluted neologisms), the ambiguities within feminisms, and the tensions and congruences between and among feminisms and postmodernisms. In this chapter I will review the genealogy of postmodernisms and describe basic concepts of postmodernity and postmodernism. As feminisms have been well examined in the nursing literature, I will describe only the various strands of postmodern feminist theories. I will then examine the commonalities and tensions among these perspectives. To illustrate how these perspectives can be used in nursing theory development, research, and practice, I will use examples of a specific women's health research problem—the effects of social policies, scientific discourses, and ideologies on maternal identity transitions for employed women (Miller, 1994, 1996).

POSTMODERNISMS/ POSTMODERNITY

Postmodernisms are difficult to define in that they refer to both a historical period and to complex, heterogeneous theoretical perspectives. Some theorists distinguish between the time period (postmodernity) and the perspectives (postmodernisms). As a period, postmodernity is "post" modernization, that is, after the period of industrialization and the birth and growth of the nation-state (Harvey, 1989). As a collection of theories, postmodernisms are far more difficult to define.

No one agrees exactly on the definition or characteristics of postmodernisms, except that they represent a reaction to or departure from modernism (Harvey, 1989; McGowan, 1991). There is no *single* postmodernism. Postmodernism*s* comprise many different areas of ontology and epistemology and represent cross-cultural intellectual movements encompassing multidisciplinary approaches to knowledges and knowledge making.

Nevertheless, these theories tend to have certain commonalities. Postmodern perspectives critique the modern concepts of self and subjectivity and challenge Enlightenment forms of the alleged neutrality of modernist science and knowledge (e.g., the "God's eye view" or "view from nowhere"; Haraway, 1991). Postmodern theories reject "grand narratives" or metatheory (Lyotard, 1984). No narratives are privileged over others; any narrative is seen as just that, one more narrative. No single theory can possibly capture the "truth" because every truth is incomplete, partial, and culture bound. Examples of the grand narratives critiqued by postmodernists include modern Western science, Marxism, Freudian psychoanalysis, and feminism.

In place of these grand narratives, or metadiscourses, postmodern theorists look for multiplicities, indeterminancies, fragmentations, and pluralities in small-scale situated knowledges. Common among many postmodernisms is the recognition of the *pluralism* of cultures, traditions, values, theories, ideologies, and forms of life. These perspectives hold that no knowledge can be assessed outside the context of the culture and the languages/symbols that make it possible and endow it with meaning (Bauman, 1992; Haraway, 1991).

Postmodernisms and Cultural Critiques

In this discussion, I will use *postmodernisms* to refer to specific forms of cultural critiques arising in academia in the mid-1970s. These are antifoundationalist critiques that are also radical in their commitment to transforming the existing Western social order (McGowan, 1991). As such, feminist theorizing, which has long proclaimed the notion of the Enlightenment Western social order to be partial, foundationalist, contingent, and historically situated, can be seen to fit with postmodernisms as a radical cultural critique (see Kaplan, 1988). Likewise, nursing science, which has developed outside the predominantly male medical establishment and has critiqued the notion of empirical knowing as the *only* way of knowing (Carper, 1978), can be an antifoundationalist critique.

Genealogies of Postmodernisms

Postmodernisms have their roots in a multiplicity of (often conflicting) European and American nineteenth- and twentieth-century philosophies and social theories. These include romanticism, relativism, Husserl's phenomenology, Nietzsche's nihilism, Sartre and de Beauvoir's existentialism, Dewey's pragmatism, Meadian symbolic interactionism, the Frankfurt school's critical social theory, and various Marxist teachings (Rosenau, 1992). However, some genealogists see postmodern perspectives more specifically arising in the 1960s and 1970s as reactions to the structuralist movement that began in the linguistics of Ferdinand de Saussure (1956) and the anthropology of Claude Lévi-Strauss (1963), who postulated that all philosophical inquiry is essentially a matter of language. (Structuralists view the human experience of the world as undergirded by a unifying structure, language. Structuralists are concerned philosophically with how meaning is constructed through language.)

This reaction against structuralism had been precipitated by historical events that provoked a "crisis" in European philosophical and political thought. Such events as the Algerian war of independence, the withdrawal of France from Vietnam and the U.S. escalation of that conflict, the Hungarian and Czechoslovakian uprisings of the late 1960s, the devastating response to those popular movements by the Soviet Communist Party, and the student uprising in Paris in 1968 caused these intellectuals to examine what they had previously understood to be "truth" and ways of knowing. They began to question both liberal humanism and Marxism (a greater influence for intellectuals in Europe than in North America), and these questions led them to examine the structures underlying Western thought (universal truth, identity, subjectivity, reason, scientific progress, and logic). They found these foundations to be sociohistoric constructions serving specific political ends, and not universal truths (Bauman, 1992; Rabine, 1988).

Derrida (1982) connected language, culture, and society and moved beyond structuralism toward poststructuralism. Both structuralists and poststructuralists see meaning as social construction, produced by arrangements of language; unlike structuralists, however, poststructuralists deny any universal system to culture and society. The poststructuralist move was rapidly taken up by a variety of academic disciplines through the theories and practices of deconstruction, semiotics, and historiography.

Postmodernisms in North America

In North America there was a concomitant crisis in philosophical and political thought brought about (for example) by increasing discouragement with the "advances" of technologies; the drawn-out military attack on Vietnam, the effects of the Vietnam war on politics, and the evidence of inhuman behavior evinced by American GIs at My Lai; and the questioning of Enlightenment values raised by the "others" in North American culture—feminists, postcolonial peoples, indigenous peoples, and persons of non-European descent.

Poststructuralisms/postmodernisms have gained increasing popularity in a variety of intellectual disciplines, including literary studies, neopragmatic philosophy, anthropology, sociology, social psychology, political science, history, geography, psychology, and feminist studies. Postmodern thought is represented by the notion of paradigm changes in the philosophy of science formulated by Kuhn (1970); developments in the "hard" sciences such as chaos theory, subatomic physics, and fractal geometry (Murphy, 1990); and the reemergence of concern in ethics, politics, and anthropology for the validity and dignity of those on the margins.

Postmodern Strategies

As the concepts representative of postmodernisms are often worded in neologisms, I include some explanations here. However, these explanations can be only tentative, as any attempt to clarify these key concepts must be, to avoid the risk of oversimplifying complex new ways of thinking. My explanations of these concepts may help the nurse reader to see how postmodern perspectives can be used in critical thinking, theorizing, and researching. It may be most useful to look at these concepts as strategies (Derrida, 1982, describes his technique of deconstruction as a "strategic device"). I will also demonstrate how I used these postmodern strategies in a specific nursing research study on women's identity transitions as they became first-time mothers.

Deconstruction. Culler (1982) describes deconstruction as a way to examine how language operates below the everyday level of consciousness in creating meanings. Derrida (1982) has developed deconstruction as a technique for challenging the *binary oppositions* (male/female, nature/culture, public/private, qualitative/quantitative) that are basic to Western Enlightenment thinking. Deconstruction challenges assumptions of opposition and hierarchy by drawing attention to the way each term in a binary pair contains elements of the other and depends on the other for its meaning. The meaning of each word is determined as much by what it is not as by what it is.

Deconstructive readings, then, rely on the gaps, inconsistencies, and contradictions in a discourse or text. By attending to these inconsistencies and marginalized meanings, the deconstructive reader can find meanings beyond those apparent in a literal reading. For the researcher, deconstructive strategies can focus attention on hidden meanings in culturally embedded metaphors (Hare-Mustin & Marecek, 1988). An example from my research work on new mothers' identity transitions would be to deconstruct the oppositions in employment/motherhood, family leave/child care, and public/private, subjecting these terms to a critical examination by looking at their historical contexts and by refusing to see them as dichotomies. Viewing employment and mothering not as an oppositional pair but as two of the many facets of women's multiple identities opens up new possibilities for researchers examining the effects of workplace and family policies on mothers' health.

Discourses. Hollway (1989) defines discourses as an "interrelated system of statements which cohere around common meanings and values" (p. 231). Weedon (1987) describes discourses as the structuring principles of a society that constitute and are reproduced in social institutions, modes of thought, and individual subjectivity. In my nursing research example, the discourses on "good" mothering include child-care books; visits to the pediatrician, obstetrician, or midwife; and representations of mothers on television and in the movies, in magazine depictions, and in advertising images. Included in these discourses are the publicly disseminated results of medical, nursing, psychological, and sociological research on bonding, child development, maternal deprivation, attachment, maternal role acquisition, salience of maternal role, and so on. These make up a body of *normalizing discourses* defining satisfactory and socially acceptable maternal-child health or development (Henriques, Hollway, Urwin, Venn, & Walkerdine, 1984).

Power/knowledge. Foucault (1980) joins knowledge and power together as power/knowledge and applies this construction to all knowledge, but especially to the knowledge production of the human sciences. Power is present in all social interactions, including the relations of researcher to researched and nurse to client. Generally (except when they are researching elites), researchers, through their position as experts, have more power than do their respondents/participants. Nurse researchers need to make every effort to reduce such power inequities in their research. However, it is also important for nurse researchers to acknowledge that the power imbalance in their research relationships is not entirely determined by those who are directly interacting; rather, like all other power relations, it is constructed by the historical sociopolitical times in which the interaction takes place. Nursing practice also contains these elements of power/knowledge, and nurses need to be aware of and sensitive to the power they hold over others' lives because of the scientific knowledge they possess.

Genealogizing. Genealogizing is a method for categorizing concepts by framing them within a historical narrative and rendering them temporally and culturally specific. For example, genealogizing maternal practices by studying the history of the family in U.S. culture, as Coontz does in *The Way We Never Were* (1992), allows researchers to see how ideologies of mothering develop in specific cultures within specific classes. Foucault (1980) calls genealogy a "history of the present." He suggests that by genealogizing family life, one can identify microsources of oppression and domination in personal life (Dreyfus & Rabinow, 1983), a concept very similar to the feminist slogan "The personal is political." All of the aforementioned strategies are used to "undo" the effects of two other concepts one finds discussed frequently in postmodern writings, universalizing and essentializing.

Universalizing. Universalizing involves making statements referring to all members of a category (e.g., woman or mother) that are transhistorical and acontextual. For example, discourses that universalize mothering practices based on idealized heterosexual European American middle-class families have marginalized and stigmatized women whose mothering is based in different cultural patterns or sexual orientations. Research conducted on lower-income African American mothers based on middle-class European American values ignores racial and economic oppression and misses explanations and interpretations arising from the historical and cultural experiences of black women in families (Joseph, 1981). Universalizing mothering as a heterosexual activity excludes the many lesbians who have chosen to bear, adopt, and/or rear children. Universalizing motherhood as a necessary identity position for a woman marginalizes those women who are infertile or who, for various reasons, choose to be childless.

Essentializing. Essentializing is the reduction of concepts to an essence, or a belief in an inherent, eternal nature. In terms of women, this defines a "female" nature that manifests itself in such characteristics as gentleness, goodness, nurturance, and sensitivity. Essentialist discourses on mothering and nurturing abound in both conservative rhetoric and sociobiological discourses, as well as in the cultural feminist discourses, where they valorize women's nurturing role (e.g., Ruddick, 1989). An example of essentializing is the tendency in some Western feminist thought to posit an essential "womanness" for all women despite racial, class, religious, sexual orientation, ethnic, or cultural differences among them (Spellman, 1988). These essentializing trends in both cultural feminism and biological determinism obscure the heterogeneity of women and prevent political analysis of heterogeneity in feminist theory.

POSTMODERN FEMINISMS AND FEMINIST POSTMODERNISMS

Some feminist scholars believe that postmodernisms can be an antidote to essentialism in feminist theorizing and research, especially on the (sometimes very different) issues of childbearing and child rearing (Spellman, 1988). Postmodern feminists argue against the notion of a unique, single feminist standpoint, which essentializes female identities. Such a standpoint is impossible from a postmodernist position because there is no Archimedean standpoint from which to view "reality" (Harding, 1990). A postmodern feminist raises the question of *which* feminist standpoint is *the* feminist standpoint: that of a European American potter who lives on a Vermont farm, that of an African American college professor teaching in New York City, that of a traditional birth attendant living in rural Pakistan, or that of a Filipina housekeeper in British Columbia? Each of these women might have different, and even multiple, feminist standpoints.

Like the postmodern philosophies, feminist theory is not a unified metatheory, but a number of theories, related by a perspective through which diverse women's needs and experiences are considered inherently valid (Klein, 1983). The many feminist theoretical and political positions currently espoused are those with liberal, Marxist, dual systems, radical, cultural, psychoanalytic, socialist, existentialist, Third World, African American, ecological, postmodern, and multiple simultaneous perspectives. Although postmodern feminists do not deny the existence of male dominance and oppression of women in a variety of situations, they also allow for the possibility that women can exert power over other women, men, and children. As hooks (1990) notes, analyses of women's capacity to dominate constitute a way to deconstruct and challenge the simplistic notion that man is the enemy and that woman is always virtuous. Postmodern feminist deconstructions of oppression and domination permit researchers and theorists to examine women's participation in the perpetuation and maintenance of systems of domination.

Although there are tensions between postmodernisms and feminisms (see below), some feminist scholars see enough parallels and convergences between the two that they call themselves postmodern feminists (Diamond & Quinby, 1988; Flax, 1990; Heckman, 1990). Epistemologically, postmodern feminists view knowledges as forms of socially negotiated and historically contextualized understandings, rather than as accurate renderings of "reality" (Harding, 1990).

Postmodern feminists acknowledge that because women's experiences vary along so many axes (age, race-ethnicity, class, sexual identification, and so on), it is impossible to describe those experiences under one theory without ignoring the significant differences among women. Just as women are not one but many, so feminisms and feminist theories must be plural, partial, multiple, contingent, local, and small-scale. Feminist postmodernists also try to avoid the privileging of one axis over another, seeking instead complex multiple locations and identities of women's lives. They acknowledge diversity among women and the possibility of the coexistence of many feminisms.

Feminisms/Postmodernisms: Mutually Corrective

Feminist postmodernists see feminisms and postmodernisms as complementary and mutually corrective (Flax, 1990; Fraser, 1989; Heckman, 1990). Feminist critiques extend the postmodern critiques of rationalism by revealing their gendered character, and postmodern critiques help feminisms to avoid universal concepts in analyses of the oppressions of women.

Like postmodernisms, feminisms are radical movements that challenge the fundamental assumptions of the modernist legacy. Feminist theorists have long argued that the Enlightenment humanist epistemologies are flawed and gender biased and must be displaced. Both movements are very concerned with language and the way language shapes and constructs "reality." Both challenge certain defining characteristics of modernism, such as the anthropocentric definition of knowledge. Historically, second-wave feminisms and postmodernisms became prominent modes of theorizing at around the same time; in fact, many feminist theorists and postmodern theorists feel that postmodern arguments are extensions of feminist arguments (Gergen, 1991; Harvey, 1989; Scott, 1988).

The very multiplicity of postmodern philosophies and strategies coincides with the diversity and multiplicity of feminist positions. Postmodern perspectives allow for a multiplicity of feminist positions, acknowledging the contradictions implicit in them and accommodating ambiguity. Postmodern feminisms avoid a unitary theory about woman and view all theories about women as incomplete, context bound, and partial.

Many postmodern feminists find congruences between the works of Michel Foucault and various feminisms. None of these feminist scholars denies that Foucault's writings are androcentric, and none denies that the intersections between feminisms and postmodernisms are filled with tension. Among the congruences these writers have cited between Foucault's works and feminisms are his overtly political program, which deals with power and resistance and which connects power and knowledge; his method of genealogy, which is used to contextualize phenomena historically and locally and to unmask all forms of "True Discourse" by determining their conditions of existence and their political effects; and the notion found in his work of the social construction of gender and sexuality (see, e.g., Diamond & Quinby, 1988).

Tensions and Conflicts

Although there are convergences and fluidities between postmodernisms and feminisms, the relationship is not without conflicts, contradictions, and tensions. Some of this is due to the ambiguities within feminisms: the conflicting strands among feminisms and between liberal and cultural feminisms, and the contradictions between feminist empiricists and standpoint feminists and between feminisms as cultural critiques and as political activisms.

A major tension exists between the social constructionist nature of postmodern thinking and the feminist essentialist fear that refusing to recognize woman as a universal class will result in women's inability to act politically. Postmodernist social constructionists feel that theorizing women's experiences as a universal category leads to an ahistorical conception of women's oppression and a suppression of differentiation among women. The essentialists feel that the weakening of essences through the social constructionist critique erodes the basis for subjectivity and solidarity among women. The essentialists fear that acting as if there is no such thing as woman as a universal class will destroy women's ability to act politically (Fuss, 1990).

Other tensions between these perspectives include the stated need for feminists to retain a sex/gender dichotomy as a concept of analysis, which clashes with postmodern thinkers' rejection of dualisms as social constructions (Scott, 1989); the androcentric nature of the work of the male spokespersons of postmodernisms, who have ignored gender in their writings; and the problematic that postmodernisms express the claims of white, privileged men questioning the Enlightenment, although women have never experienced an Enlightenment.

Responding to Unresolved Tensions

Although these tensions remain unresolved, some feminist postmodernists have suggested ways to live with these contradictions. Feminists can recognize the contradictions within/between feminisms and postmodernisms and embrace them, adopting positions that are tolerant of ambiguity. Feminists can also take the critical deconstructive insights of postmodernisms and harness them to a progressive and substantive feminist politics. Fuss (1990) suggests not taking sides in an essentialist/constructionist debate, but instead problematizing the binary form of opposition of essentialism/constructionism, recognizing the plurality of different essentialisms, and using essentialisms as a tool for displacement, interruption, and resistance. Feminist postmodernists can also take up positions as contextual pragmatists, taking what is useful from postmodernisms while adhering to their own political agenda (Seigfried, 1993).

WHAT POSTMODERN FEMINIST PERSPECTIVES OFFER NURSES

I suggest that nurses become contextual pragmatists by critically evaluating individual instances in which feminist postmodern perspectives offer innovative, complex lenses through which to view the various truths around them. Postmodern feminist philosophies and epistemologies can be valuable perspectives for the ongoing process of developing the nursing sciences. They are particularly valuable in the way they encourage nurses to attend to ontological and political assumptions regarding knowledge, language, and power in social scientific research, knowledge, and practice. In researching women's health, feminist postmodern researchers would seek to avoid totalizing women's diverse experiences on the basis of one ethnic, social, economic, or political group. They would look beyond the surface similarities of a mythical woman's voice and develop multiple paradigms that attend to the wide diversity of real women's experiences along multiple axes of existence. They would question who has gained by the status quo of the research act, who has been excluded from research opportunities, as well as what the effects of being involved in research might have on the research participants, the research findings, and the researcher.

Foucault's concept of normalizing discourses is especially relevant for nurses to apply to the ways power operates in postmodern times. The power/knowledge concept directly addresses the normalizing disciplines of the human sciences (including nursing), in which experts (including nurses) dictate to women how they should be and which marginalize those women who fail to meet their standards (Allen, Allman, & Powers, 1991). Postmodern feminist perspectives allow nursing scientists and practitioners to see past the proscriptive normalizing discourses of predetermined female roles to the rapidly changing multiplicities, ambiguities, and indeterminacies of identity shifts and transformations in the postmodern world.

In theory development for the nursing sciences, feminist postmodern perspectives can be utilized to challenge and resist dominant received knowledges and to generate alternative knowledges based on human lived experiences. In my own work on mothering practices of employed women, I attempted to produce a small-scale, situated microtheory based on *some* mothers' practices, their understandings, and the meanings they made out of a changing world (Miller, 1994, 1996). This partial theory stands in contrast to the grand metanarratives of current feminist mothering theories, which often serve as normalizing discourses by which mothers judge themselves and are judged by others. No single mothering theory can possibly capture the "truth" about all mothers, as every truth is incomplete, partial, and culture bound. This research adds to specific, local knowledges that inform and lead to understanding and to change. Such microtheories are useful for addressing questions of how social power is exercised and how social relationships, especially of gender, may be transformed (see Diamond & Quinby, 1988).

Dickson (1990) uses postmodern feminist perspectives to analyze women's lived experiences with menopause in relationship to the power(ful)/knowledge of the current scientific/medical discourses. By developing this "alternative knowledge of menopause," Dickson reveals how truth is interpreted and how assumptions and values affect what is viewed as knowledge. Developing theories that emerge from knowledge generated by those experiencing a phenomenon challenges accepted ways of thinking and uncovers the resistances to power structures in women's lives. Practitioners can then use this knowledge of resistance to work with women in cocreating and transforming the knowledges and ideologies that shape dominant discourses.

Discoveries made by feminist postmodern nurse scientists will lead to changes in practice. Critically combining postmodern and feminist perspectives will help nurses caring for real clients who live messy, contingent, arbitrary, and complex lives. For example, a nurse who is aware of feminist postmodern critiques of normalizing discourses will be sensitive to her power and will avoid judgmental statements that may force dichotomizing choices on women in transition. Assumptions of heterosexuality (saying to a lesbian client, "I hope you're using condoms"), age or developmentally appropriate actions ("Well, what do you expect, you are 47!" to a woman discussing her vaginal dryness), physical limitations ("You're taking up skydiving at your age?"), and ethnically "normalized" behaviors ("Well, I suppose you're keeping this baby," to a pregnant Latina teen) are all normalizing discourses that discount the differences among individual women trying to make sense of their own experiences.

Watson (1995) notes that it is imperative that nurses be aware of and keep up with the rapidly changing philosophies and theories that reflect today's fragmented times. She goes further to suggest that "nursing, like all other disciplines, must now yield to a postmodern approach" (p. 63). I would like to add to this injunction by suggesting that feminist nursing scientists and practitioners should now join their colleagues in the other social sciences and practice disciplines by critically combining postmodern perspectives with their feminist perspectives.

REFERENCES

Allen, D. G., Allman, K. K. M., & Powers, P. (1991). Feminist nursing research without gender. *Advances in Nursing Science, 13*(3), 49-58.

Anderson, J. M. (1991). Current directions in nursing research: Toward a poststructuralist and feminist epistemology. *Canadian Journal of Nursing Research, 23*(3), 1-7.

Bauman, Z. (1992). *Intimations of postmodernity.* London: Routledge.

Bernstein, R. J. (1983). *Beyond objectivism and relativism: Science, hermeneutics, and praxis.* Philadelphia: University of Pennsylvania Press.

Bunting, S., & Campbell, J. C. (1990). Feminism and nursing: Historical perspectives. *Advances in Nursing Science, 12*(4), 11-24.

Carper, B. A. (1978). Fundamental patterns of knowing in nursing. *Advances in Nursing Science, 1*(1), 13-23.

Coontz, S. (1992). *The way we never were: American families and the nostalgia trap.* New York: Basic Books.

Culler, J. (1982). *On deconstruction: Theory and criticism after structuralism.* Ithaca, NY: Cornell University Press.

Derrida, J. (1982). *Margins of philosophy* (A. Bass, Trans.). Chicago: University of Chicago Press.

Diamond, I., & Quinby, L. (Eds.). (1988). *Feminism and Foucault: Reflections of resistance.* Boston: Northeastern University Press.

Dickson, G. L. (1990). A feminist poststructuralist analysis of the knowledge of menopause. *Advances in Nursing Science, 12*(3), 15-31.

Doering, L. (1992). Power and knowledge in nursing: A feminist poststructuralist view. *Advances in Nursing Science, 14*(4), 24-33.

Dreyfus, H. L., & Rabinow, P. (1983). *Michel Foucault: Beyond structuralism and hermeneutics.* Chicago: The University of Chicago Press.

Dzurec, L. C. (1989). The necessity for and evolution of multiple paradigms for nursing research: A poststructuralist perspective. *Advances in Nursing Science, 11*(4), 69-77.

Flax, J. (1990). *Thinking fragments: Psychoanalysis, feminism, and postmodernism in the contemporary West.* Berkeley: University of California Press.

Foucault, M. (1980). *Power/knowledge* (C. Gordon, L. Marshall, J. Mepham, & K. Soper, Trans.). New York: Pantheon.

Fraser, N. (1989). *Unruly practices: Power, discourse, and gender in contemporary social theory.* Minneapolis: University of Minnesota Press.

Fuss, D. (1990). *Essentially speaking: Feminism, nature, and difference.* London: Routledge.

Gergen, K. J. (1991). *The saturated self: Dilemmas of identity in contemporary life.* New York: Basic Books.

Haraway, D. J. (1991). Situated knowledges: The science question in feminism and the privilege of partial perspective. In D. J. Haraway, *Simians, cyborgs, and women: The reinvention of nature* (pp. 183-201). New York: Routledge.

Harding, S. (1990). Feminism, science, and the anti-Enlightenment critiques. In L. J. Nicholson (Ed.), *Feminism/postmodernism* (pp. 83-106). New York: Routledge.

Hare-Mustin, R. T., & Marecek, J. (1988). The meaning of gender difference: Gender theory, postmodernism and psychology. *American Psychologist, 43,* 455-464.

Harvey, D. (1989). *The condition of postmodernity.* Oxford, UK: Basil Blackwell.

Heckman, S. J. (1990). *Gender and knowledge: Elements of a postmodern feminism.* Boston: Northeastern University Press.

Henriques, J., Hollway, W., Urwin, C., Venn, C., & Walkerdine, V. (1984). *Changing the subject: Psychology, social regulation and subjectivity.* London: Methuen.

Hollway, W. (1989). *Subjectivity and method in psychology: Gender, meaning and science.* London: Sage.

hooks, b. (1990). Feminism: A transformational politics. In D. L. Rhode (Ed.), *Theoretical perspectives on sexual difference* (pp. 185-197). New Haven, CT: Yale University Press.

Joseph, G. I. (1981). Black mothers and daughters: Their roles and functions in American society. In G. I. Joseph & J. Lewis (Eds.), *Common differences: Conflicts in black and white feminist perspectives* (pp. 75-126). Boston: South End.

Kaplan, E. A. (Ed.). (1988). *Postmodernism and its discontents.* London: Verso.

Klein, R. D. (1983). How to do what we want to do: Thoughts about feminist methodology. In G. Bowles & R. D. Klein (Eds.), *Theories of women's studies* (pp. 88-104). Boston: Routledge & Kegan Paul.

Kuhn, T. (1970). *The structure of scientific revolutions* (2nd ed.). Chicago: University of Chicago Press.

Lévi-Strauss, C. (1963). *Structural anthropology* (C. Jacobson & B. G. Schoepf, Trans.). New York: Basic Books.

Lister, P. (1991). Approaching models of nursing from a postmodernist perspective. *Journal of Advanced Nursing, 16,* 206-212.

Lyotard, J.-F. (1984). *The postmodern condition: A report on knowledge* (G. Bennington & B. Massumi, Trans.). Minneapolis: University of Minnesota Press.

McGowan, J. (1991). *Postmodernism and its critics.* Ithaca, NY: Cornell University Press.

Miller, S. (1994). *Improvising identities: Career reentry for new mothers.* Unpublished doctoral dissertation. University of California, San Francisco.

Miller, S. (1996). Questioning, acquiescing, balancing, resisting: Strategies for identity improvisations for career committed new mothers. *Health Care for Women International, 17,* 109-131.

Murphy, N. (1990). Scientific realism and postmodern philosophy. *British Journal for the Philosophy of Science, 41*, 291-303.

Rabine, L. W. (1988). A feminist politics of non-identity. *Feminist Studies, 14*(1), 11-31.

Rosenau, P. R. (1992). *Postmodernism and the social sciences: Insights, inroads, and intrusions.* Princeton, NJ: Princeton University Press.

Ruddick, S. (1989). *Maternal thinking.* Boston: Beacon.

Saussure, F. de. (1956). *A course in general linguistics* (W. Baskin, Trans.). New York: Philosophical Library.

Scott, J. (1989). Gender: A useful category of historical analysis. In E. Weed (Ed.), *Coming to terms* (pp. 81-101). New York: Routledge.

Scott, J. W. (1988). Deconstructing equality-versus-difference: The uses of poststructuralist theory for feminism. *Feminist Studies, 14*(1), 32-51.

Seigfried, C. H. (1993). Shared communities of interest: Feminism and pragmatism. *Hypatia, 8*(2), 1-14.

Spellman, E. (1988). *Inessential woman.* Boston: Beacon.

Thompson, J. L. (1985). Practical discourses about nursing: Going beyond empiricism and historicism. *Advances in Nursing Science, 7*(4), 59-71.

Watson, J. (1995). Postmodernism and knowledge development in nursing. *Nursing Science Quarterly, 8*(2), 60-64.

Weedon, C. (1987). *Feminist practice and poststructuralist theory.* Oxford, UK: Basil Blackwell.

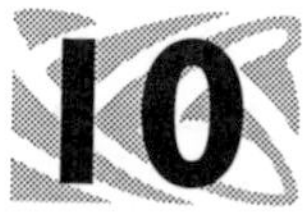

Consciousness-Raising as a Feminist Nursing Action

Promise and Practice, Present and Future

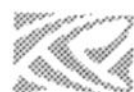

DOROTHY J. HENDERSON

Over the past 25 years, increasing numbers of nurse scholars have viewed their domain through the lens of feminist or critical social theories. Although feminist and critical perspectives have most commonly been suggested as methodologies for nursing research or for framing women's health issues, their application to nursing practice is quite recent (Hagedorn, 1995; Kendall, 1992; Moccia, 1988; Sampselle, 1991; Stevens & Hall, 1992; Thompson, 1991; Woods, 1995). These latest applications have wrestled with the method of feminist nursing practice and have included various suggestions for feminist nursing actions. Whereas a few have proposed political action as the method of activity (Moccia, 1988), most have recommended some form of consciousness-raising as a primary nursing action for feminist/emancipatory nursing practice. Consciousness-raising has been presented as an ideal method of applying feminist principles (such as nonhierarchical power relations and linking the personal and the political) to emancipatory nursing practice. To promote a more thorough understanding of consciousness-raising and its relationship to feminist emancipatory nursing practice, I explore in this chapter the roots of consciousness-raising, including the concepts of enlightenment, empowerment, and emancipation. I also review here the application of consciousness-raising in emancipatory nursing practice, employing examples from recent literature as well as from my own experience as a feminist nurse. I use these examples to explore some problems with both the promise and practice of consciousness-raising and to discuss the future of consciousness-raising as a feminist nursing action.

CONSCIOUSNESS-RAISING

Consciousness may be defined as the quality or state of being aware, especially of something within oneself, but also of external objects, states, or facts. *Consciousness-raising,* a concept rooted in feminist and critical political movements and writings, refers to the process of increasing the state or quality of being aware, particularly as it applies to issues of personal and political freedom. Within these frameworks, consciousness-raising has generally been defined as an educational engagement in which people recognize and articulate the social, political, economic, and personal constraints on their freedom and become empowered to take action to remove those constraints.

According to the critical social theorist Paulo Freire (1970/1990), consciousness-raising involves a critical and liberating dialogue in which individuals discover the power imbalances within a society that contribute to their oppression, as well as the hidden distortions within themselves that help to maintain an oppressive society. As a Brazilian activist and educator, Freire locates this dialogue between oppressed peasants, who contribute the empirical, experiential knowledge of their lives, and revolutionary leaders, who contribute the theoretical analysis of that experience. In his work there are relatively clear lines separating the oppressed, who are illiterate peasants; the oppressors, who are the ruling class; and the revolutionary leaders, who are invested in improving the lives of the oppressed. Freire emphasizes the elimination of class differences through radical teaching methods in literacy campaigns.

In contrast to Freire's Marxist class analysis, early feminist consciousness-raising groups focused on power imbalances based on gender and advocated the personalization of women's experience of oppression. Women were urged to look to their shared experiences to develop their understanding and a course of action. However, women were reminded that their experiences could not be limited to the personal, but rather illuminated the experiences of all women (Rosenthal, 1984).

In a further break with Freire's work, feminist consciousness-raising groups blurred the line between leader (holder of theoretical knowledge) and oppressed (holder of experiential knowledge). There was no distinction between theoreticians and experientialists; everyone had the opportunity for analytic and empirical input (MacKinnon, 1989). Feminist consciousness-raising affirms the self as knower of the self's condition, while at the same time critiquing the conditions that have created that self; everyone becomes a theorist. As bell hooks (1992) describes it, "When our lived experience of theorizing is fundamentally linked to processes of self-recovery, of collective liberation, no gap exists between theory and practice" (p. 80). In feminist consciousness-raising, the distinction between knowledge labeled "theory" and knowledge labeled "experience" is a false dichotomy.

Notwithstanding these differences, both Freirean and early feminist consciousness-raising have several features in common. Consciousness is raised in relatively homogeneous groups of individuals, who talk about a shared sense of reality and a shared sense of oppression. In so doing, those engaged recognize their problems as group problems rather than as individual problems (MacKinnon, 1989). They come to see the ways they have internalized the dominant view of their inferiority and thus may have contributed to their oppressive life situations. Ironically, an increased awareness of complicity in their own oppression can lead to a greater sense of individual empowerment, as they recognize that they both shape and are shaped by their reality. Ideally, the awareness of their own ability to change their situation leads to active efforts to do so, which can lead to change in the greater social fabric.

Thus, within both perspectives, consciousness-raising is proposed as an individual and a group experience. It can contribute to psychological change for the individual and to social transformation for groups and communities. Fonow and Cook (1991) emphasize the importance of both personal and political outcomes of consciousness-raising as "emotional catharsis, academic insight and intellectual product, and increasing politicization and activism" (p. 3). This process occurs in a tripartite, overlapping experience of enlightenment, empowerment, and emancipation. Each of these exists in dynamic relation to the others.

ENLIGHTENMENT, EMPOWERMENT, AND EMANCIPATION

When conducting women's issues groups with women who were in treatment for substance abuse and eating disorders, I showed a film that exposed the images of women in advertising in the United States. The women began to see the ways in which their negative attitudes about their bodies, their abilities, and their relationships with other women might be based on messages in the media, and not on their personal inadequacy. In discussions after the film, women commented that they would never look at magazine or television advertisements featuring the perfect female in the same way as before. They were angry at being sold a bill of goods about the inadequacy of their own bodies and abilities. After this incident, some of the women began to challenge the norm of women as being a certain body type, wearing makeup, and being sex symbols for consumer products. These challenges took the shape of personal lifestyle changes and public demonstrations. Enlightenment, empowerment, and emancipation had occurred.

In consciousness-raising, *enlightenment* is the experience of coming to see oneself and one's place in society in a radically new way. This occurs when connections are made between others with similar experiences in a way that encourages self-reflection and analysis (Fay, 1987; Freire, 1970/1990; Lather, 1991). The analysis develops out of, but is not limited to, theory, such as feminist and critical theories. In the previous example, the women experienced enlightenment when they saw the film and discussed similar experiences with other women in the discussions after viewing.

Empowerment is the process by which a group of individuals become galvanized to act on their own behalf (Gibson, 1991; Kieffer, 1984; Lather, 1991). It is also a state of feeling more powerful than previously, of feeling one has the ability to affect others and to change social institutions. Empowerment is an interpersonal and intrapersonal experience, with each contributing to the other. After watching the film, the women became empowered as they discussed their common experience and felt capable of doing something to improve their condition. Often, shared anger combined with a beginning expression of self-regard or love are key motivators in empowerment.

Emancipation is both the process and the state of liberation (Fay, 1987; Freire, 1970/1990; Lather, 1991). People learn who they are and gain the collective power to determine the direction of their lives. The nature of emancipation is dynamic. Because human beings cannot be separated from their social and historical contexts, reality is not a static entity but a process—a transformation. By engaging in acts of enlightenment and empowerment, human beings become liberated—become more fully human. In the groups that saw the film described above, emancipation occurred when the women described feeling that they had choices about wearing makeup or purchasing body-altering products. Taking steps to change that condition for other women, such as protesting the use of women as sex objects in advertising, is another example of an emancipatory moment.

Although the preceding discussion presents enlightenment, empowerment, and emancipation as though they exist in a distinct and linear relationship, this is not the case. For some women in the example, recognizing the ways their negative self-images had been shaped by the media was enlightening, empowering, and emancipating all at once. People often experience enlightenment, empowerment, and emancipation as overlapping circles of insight and action that create and are the result of raised consciousness. For others, empowerment and emancipation occurred simultaneously as they staged protests about a local billboard that used a partially clad woman to advertise vodka (the billboard was finally removed).

CONSCIOUSNESS-RAISING IN NURSING PRACTICE

Consciousness-raising has been suggested as a method of nursing practice by both feminist and critical social theorists in nursing. Sampselle (1991) calls upon nurses to prevent violence against women by using a feminist practice base. She details several nursing actions that "can empower women . . . by raising the consciousness of their clients" (p. 485). These include pointing out to clients offensive images of women in advertising, placing health care issues within historical and social context, and using language and actions that affirm women as equal partners in their health care.

Like Moccia (1988), whose activist agenda for nurses focuses on the social policy level, Kendall (1992) recommends emancipatory nursing actions that are broader in scope than Sampselle's. Kendall calls for actions that "increase the potential for oppressed groups to take power from those that oppress them, including fighting for a national health insurance policy, an increase in funding for the homeless, or a change in the political power base of an organization" (p. 9). Kendall does refer, though indirectly, to consciousness-raising in her description of one such action: "helping to empower politically and socially disenfranchised groups by providing alternative and critical explanations for their situations" (p. 9). Stevens and Hall (1992) recommend similar actions within a community health nursing practice, offering the example of nurses' engaging in critical dialogue with a community group. They suggest that nurses take a stand against oppressive conditions that damage health, engage in critical dialogue with communities, and act with communities for change.

Although few nurses have reported on experiences of consciousness-raising as nursing action, three recent reports of feminist participatory action research projects have included detailed descriptions of consciousness-raising (Hagedorn, 1995; Henderson, 1995a; Sieng & Thompson, 1992; Thompson, 1991). Although in these cases consciousness-raising occurred in research rather than strictly practice settings, the nature of participatory research is such that practice and research are not as compartmentalized as in more traditional research methodologies (Henderson, 1995a). As with the relationship between the revolutionary leader and the oppressed, the line between practice and research is blurred. One of the important principles of consciousness-raising is the restructuring of such traditional hierarchies. Theories and practices that have been locked into linear, dualistic structures are exploded as simplistic and exploitative.

Hagedorn (1995) included consciousness-raising as one of the components in an activist nursing inquiry into young women's experience of menarche. A group of "co-researchers," three nurses and seven adolescent African American and European American women, met in a group for 8 months to explore their experiences of menarche; to review educational materials on menarche; to develop, implement, and analyze a questionnaire about menarche; and to create a 27-minute film about menarche to be used as a consciousness-raising tool with adolescent girls. In addition, the women used research into the process of the group to develop a theoretical framework for activist primary caring.

Hagedorn's work clearly illustrates the components of consciousness-raising as a feminist nursing action. The group was made up of co-researchers and was without a specific leader. A feminist process (based on Wheeler & Chinn, 1991) was used as a theory to guide the action. The group members experienced enlightenment, empowerment, and emancipation. Individual and group change occurred, and the production of the film indicates the effort made to create lasting social change.

In a similar vein, I have described feminist consciousness-raising as a nursing action with women in a drug treatment program (Henderson, 1995a). The consciousness-raising group took place within a participatory research project designed to create an all-women's treatment program in a coed therapeutic drug treatment community and to explore the experience of women going through the program. A group of eight women, myself included, of differing backgrounds and ethnicities met for 8 months to explore the ways in which our commonalities and differences could be used to create a healing environment for women in drug treatment. Numerous examples of enlightenment, empowerment, and emancipation took place within the group. Group members came to new understandings of what it means to be a woman, helped each other take risks to improve our lives and those of other women, and ultimately created an all-women's program that resulted in a different treatment experience for women and more positions for women staff.

It is important to note that in the reports of both the projects described by Hagedorn and myself, differences among the group members are glossed over. Although the groups were all women, they were both heterogeneous in terms of race and class, and Hagedorn's group members ranged in age from 13 to 50 years. In the published reports, both groups are referred to in the collective, as though there were no power imbalances inherent in the race and class differences. Hagedorn (1995) makes one reference to the conflicts posed by these differences, but immediately disclaims it and does not elaborate: "While issues of power, race and class proved to be divisive in the group process, power was shared by the co-researchers most invested in the activist primary care nursing inquiry" (pp. 6-7). We are not told which co-researchers were most invested. Similarly, in my report I describe the visible differences among the group members, but make no further mention of conflicts that arose in the group. In a telling indication of how the power imbalances played out in the projects, neither Hagedorn nor I report our own consciousness-raising experiences except as they were part of the group process.

In an earlier work, Thompson (1991) describes a feminist participatory project with Cambodian refugee women. The project was located in a combined framework of community mental health nursing and feminist participatory research methodology. Three women, a Cambodian refugee and two white community mental health nurses, codirected a group of 12 to 16 Cambodian refugee women that functioned as both a support group and a site of research. The purpose of the research was to explore the psychosocial adjustment of the refugee women in the United States and the cultural traditions that influenced their adjustment. Although Thompson describes the method of research and practice in the group process as consciousness-raising, she does not include specific explication of the consciousness-raising experience of either the Cambodian women or the coleaders in the group. However, in a later article about the project, consciousness-raising is the main theme (Sieng & Thompson, 1992). The article comprises the self-reflections of two of the project's codirectors—Sieng, a Cambodian woman who served as interpreter for the participatory project, and Thompson. Sieng begins by narrating the story of her migration to the United States and her place in the group as an interpreter. Sieng's consciousness was raised as she gained insights into the struggles of Cambodian refugee women in this country and made connections between their lives and hers. Tellingly, she moves between the pronouns *they* and *we* when describing her perceptions of Cambodian refugee women—for example: "Even if the women have good English, they still have a hard time growing accustomed to and learning this new culture. It is not only a language barrier or culture shock that we have to deal with" (Sieng & Thompson, 1992, p. 131). The text of Sieng's section of the article includes several lines in Cambodian. Clearly, Sieng's consciousness-raising occurred as she saw commonalities between the struggles of other Cambodian women and her own.

In contrast with Sieng, Thompson's consciousness was raised as she became increasingly aware of her difference from the refugee women. Labeling her experience in the group as a "powerful ground of learning," Thompson describes a number of insights she had as a white, non-Khmer-speaking, Western feminist attempting to engage in feminist process with the refugees, many of whom spoke no English (Sieng & Thompson, 1992, p. 135). She became aware of her sense of responsibility, as a U.S. citizen, for the Cambodian women's displacement. She recognized the significance of the language imbalance and the importance of learning Khmer if she was to continue working with them, and she made a commitment to learn more about the Cambodian culture and to engage more directly in efforts to improve the lives of refugee women. By including her own consciousness-raising, Thompson (and Sieng) explores more fully the power imbalances between her and the other women in the group.

THE PROMISE AND PRACTICE OF CONSCIOUSNESS-RAISING AS FEMINIST NURSING ACTION

At its core, consciousness-raising is a method of seeking and producing knowledge. The process of enlightenment, empowerment, and emancipation is the process of uncovering distortions of knowledge, creating new knowledge, and acting on that new knowledge to create individual and social change. Within a feminist nursing perspective, this production of knowledge can lead to healing, as individuals and societies recognize and overturn patterns of behavior that are destructive to health. The issue of power is inextricably linked to the pursuit and production of knowledge. As knowledge is created and identified in consciousness-raising groups, a series of questions are posed and answered within a dynamic of power relationships: What constitutes knowledge? Who decides what knowledge is valid? Who is served by this knowledge?

Differences Based on Social Constructions of Identity

Earlier models of consciousness-raising emphasized the homogeneity of the group members. Indeed, homogeneity was a contributing factor in the process of enlightenment, as individuals were able to hear their own stories in the stories of others. The power differences in these early models were located outside the group. In Freire's model, the oppressors—members of the ruling class—were not members of the consciousness-raising group. In feminist models, men were not members of the group. The challenge of today's feminists against the unity and universalism of women or of a particular class compels us to acknowledge the varying levels of power and privilege within one group.

Society confers differing degrees of power and privilege upon individuals based on the social construction of their identities. All women have not had the same experience of oppression. Beyond sexism, racism and heterosexism result in marked differences in the levels of material comforts, opportunities, and life experiences for women of color and for lesbians. As white women feminists come to acknowledge the ways we have benefited by the oppression of women of color (such as in job and housing opportunities), we have to ask if consciousness-raising as we have understood it can occur in groups of women of multiple identities. How does consciousness-raising occur when the oppressor is located not outside the group, but within the group, within ourselves?

The consciousness-raising group in which I participated was made up of women of multiple identities—of differing races and educational and class backgrounds. However, the terms *multiple* and *difference* are not specific enough. They do not convey a hierarchy of power and privilege, with some people benefiting from the losses of others. As a white, middle-class, academic woman, I found my consciousness raised as I encountered my own assumptions about race and class and my difficulty in admitting to or letting go of those assumptions. In a complex sequence of events and awarenesses during my involvement in the consciousness-raising group, I realized the absolute interdependency of race and gender in this society and in my perceptions.

On one occasion, I spoke up to protect the interests of our group when the black male director halted our decision to go forward with the women's program. During the group interaction that ensued, in which I was particularly vocal, the black woman codirector of the program was noticeably silent. When the group ended with the director's views holding sway, I reached out and patted the codirector's arm and told her it was okay. I felt that we had had a good discussion and that she shouldn't be too upset about the outcome. When she and I talked about the meeting a few weeks later, however, she told me that she felt my intervention was condescending and that she found my pat on her arm to be patronizing. She was upset that I had challenged the authority of the director in front of the other women—in essence, disrespecting him. I had assumed that she did not speak because she did not know what to say. I had thought she needed my assistance and had not considered other reasons for her remaining quiet. In reflecting on that same event, I also saw that I had less difficulty confronting the African American male director of the program than I would have had confronting a white male. Race allowed me to put less value in his authority and to challenge him with greater impunity.

In writing about my actions from the advantage of hindsight, I find myself wondering how I could have been so unaware, but in the moment I believed I was acting from a genuine effort to do the right thing. To complicate matters further, I also believe in hindsight that the codirector was truly disappointed in the outcome of the meeting and that the director was threatened by the solidarity that had taken place among the women in the group and made his decision in part because of that threat. That experience and other similar ones have led me to wonder whether it is possible to have consciousness-raising groups as they were once defined. If so, around which identities should they be constructed? As we consider whether consciousness-raising groups can take place in groups that are heterogeneous, we need to rethink the concepts of enlightenment, empowerment, and emancipation. The term *enlighten,* for example, equates light with knowledge and darkness with ignorance. This calls up colonialist images of the "white man's burden" of bringing light and truth to the dark savages.

Our knowledge of multiple identities based on differing levels of power and privilege calls into question the possibility of enlightenment, empowerment, and emancipation in consciousness-raising groups. And beyond the now-familiar critique of the use of the term *empowerment* to imply something one can instill in others (rather than something that exists within them), group heterogeneity adds a new dimension to the term. In a group of black and white women, for example, white women may find their consciousness raised about their own racism as much as about their shared experience of sexism with black women. If empowerment is the feeling of having power and being able to effect change in others, what happens when your awareness means that you feel you have had too much power to effect change in others? What if you become aware of the way you and your ancestors have contributed to the oppression of others? Others have documented necessary but painful consciousness-raising experiences such as these, which can leave an individual feeling "threatened to the core" (Frankenberg, 1993; Pratt, 1984; Reagon, 1983, p. 356). Similarly, we must reexamine the concept of emancipation in relation to groups that are racially diverse, or with mixtures of gay and straight people. The history of oppression of people of color and gays and lesbians by people of the dominant culture must make us skeptical about the possibility of achieving emancipation for or with each other in mixed groups.

Differences Based on Levels of Knowledge

The issue of power differences is also confronted in consciousness-raising groups between those who presumably possess theoretical knowledge and those who possess experiential knowledge. Although feminist consciousness-raising groups are based on the idea that everyone is both theorist and experientialist, the reality of practice is that some members of a consciousness-raising group come equipped with a feminist analysis (they are the ones who call it a consciousness-raising group, for example) and some are the recipients of that feminist analysis. Indeed, if everyone had an understanding of how they are oppressed, how they have contributed to their oppression, and what to do about it, there would be no need for consciousness-raising groups.

This imbalance between theorists and experientialists is a crucial issue for emancipatory nursing practice. Nurses do not come to the consciousness-raising group as equal players to learn together about experience and theory. Our professional status means that the consciousness-raising groups in which we engage are more closely akin to the Freirean model of the revolutionary leader with the peasants than to the feminist model, where there is no distinction between leader and peasant. Nurses are professionals with an expert level of knowledge. As such, we must be accountable for our practice. We engage in actions in pursuit of certain outcomes that are related to the health of individuals. As feminist nurses, we base our actions on an emancipatory analysis of the health issues being addressed. When we choose consciousness-raising as a means of practice with a group of individuals, we are already engaging in a hierarchical situation. Often we are the only ones to bring the critical or feminist approach to the group. I worked with women in need of drug treatment, Thompson worked with Cambodian refugee women who were in need of community mental health services, and Hagedorn worked with teens who were in need of education about menarche. Although not denying the respect that each of us afforded the women with whom we worked, it is clear that we all imparted a feminist perspective to our groups. Endeavoring to conduct groups in a nonhierarchical, respectful manner does not mean we eliminate the power imbalance that stems from our position as the holders of the theoretical knowledge, or our accountability for that position.

Perhaps because he articulates a relatively clearly delineated line between those with theoretical knowledge and those with experiential knowledge, Freire (1970/1990) is also clear about the tendency on the part of theoreticians to hold colonial and missionary attitudes toward the peasants. He reminds us of the importance of rigorous self-examination and urges us to ask ourselves these questions: "How can I dialogue if I always project ignorance onto others and never perceive my own? How can I dialogue if I consider myself a member of the in-group, the owners of truth and knowledge, for whom all nonmembers are 'these people'?" (p. 78).

I found that engaging in feminist consciousness-raising did not relieve me of having to ask Freire's questions of myself. As the sole overt feminist in the group I have described, I had a theoretical analysis of what the problem was and an agenda about how to achieve the solution. My perspective was not shared by many of the other women in the group. Although the primary task of the group was to plan the women's program, a secondary task was to identify the ways in which women's use of drugs and their recovery process are related to the gender, racial/ethnic, and social class inequalities in U.S. society; to challenge those inequalities with the group members; and to make changes in the women's lives based on those challenges. I introduced and maintained this secondary task. I found myself analyzing situations from a feminist perspective and often interjecting that perspective into the group dynamics, both in the group and in the larger program.

In part, both nursing and feminism consist of creating change in others by imparting a superior knowledge from us to them. Feminists and nurses make an effort to reduce the hierarchy in the relationship with the other, but the very need to create change through consciousness-raising implies that the other is defective in some way and needs to be changed. It is important that we not minimize this element of our work as we engage in emancipatory nursing practice. The tendency toward missionary zeal and myopia is very real. It is too easy to gloss over the power differences between the nurse professional and other group members. By raising our awareness of this hierarchy, we can explore and perhaps reduce our tendency to engage in one-way interactions.

By acknowledging our position of power in consciousness-raising groups, we can diminish power differences by reflecting on and recognizing the ways in which our own consciousnesses have been raised. Thompson, for example, describes coming to an awareness of her own complicity in the displacement of Cambodian refugees while working with the Cambodian women. At times we will find ourselves confronting our own racism, colonialism, and stereotypes. Recognizing these and bringing them to the surface can be the first steps toward our emancipation from them. Addressing issues of power and difference between group members based on identities and on location of knowledge helps us to look at the questions of who decides the validity of knowledge and who is served by knowledge. The third important question we should ask ourselves as we engage in the production of knowledge through consciousness-raising is, What constitutes knowledge?

Knowledge as Contextual, Emotional, and Embodied

Returning to the original definition offered above of consciousness-raising as an educational engagement that allows people to recognize and act to eliminate oppression, I now want to consider more carefully the concept of consciousness. What knowledge is produced as individuals share and view their life experiences through a feminist or critical lens? What are the sources of that knowledge?

From both feminist and Freirean perspectives, the knowledge produced in consciousness-raising is not disconnected from, but must be based on, the experience of the knower. Knowledge is grounded in a particular life context, in bodies, in families, in communities, in culture, and in time. As such, consciousness becomes more than the dictionary definition of being aware of something within oneself or external to oneself. In other words, consciousness is not located outside of or separate from the act of knowing. Consciousness is experience as well as the awareness of experience. MacKinnon (1989) describes this seemingly circular process as "women experiencing how they experience themselves" (p. 96). Thus knowledge produced in consciousness-raising is experiential and contextual.

How do we become conscious of, come to know, our experience in the act of consciousness-raising? How do we share our experiences with others and come to new awarenesses within ourselves based on others' sharing? My own experience has led me to conceptualize consciousness-raising more broadly than verbal interchange and to understand the knowing that occurs as more than a cognitive event. The body and the emotions are both valid sources of knowledge in consciousness-raising; such knowledge is in need of further examination.

The emotions are a critical element in the process of consciousness-raising. Although emotions are clearly connected to cognitive processes, they need to be singled out and identified as a source of knowledge, in part because of the historical valorizing of reason and rational processes as the source of true knowledge. The importance of emotions as a component of knowledge and as part of the knowledge validation process has been noted by a number of feminist and critical scholars (Collins, 1990; hooks & West, 1991; Jaggar & Bordo, 1989; MacKinnon, 1989; Narayan, 1989). Emotions have been viewed both as a source of knowledge corrupted by oppression and as a source of opposition to that oppression (Collins, 1990; Fisher, 1987).

In feminist consciousness-raising, the emotions become a means of knowing that challenges the social conditioning of the dominant culture. Emotions that do not seem to make sense on the surface may "bring to consciousness our 'gut level' awareness" that things are not as they seem, allowing us to examine hidden distortions from a critical perspective (Jaggar & Bordo, 1989, p. 161). One of the energizing emotions that often emerges as we uncover distortions and that fuels empowerment actions is anger. However, anger alone does not empower or emancipate. Freire (1970/1990) and others emphasize that love is at the core of human empowerment and resistance to oppression (Collins, 1990; hooks & West, 1991). Furthermore, love of self is a crucial ingredient in the progress toward self-determination and emancipation. Freire describes the collective experience of critical dialogue as a true act of love between people, without which emancipation is impossible.

Knowing in consciousness-raising also occurs in the body. In Western science, the body has been viewed as the enemy of objective knowing, something to be overcome if one is to perceive reality accurately. The mind is the place of knowing, and the mind has been positioned as separate from and over the body, which has been "notoriously and ubiquitously associated with the female" (Jaggar & Bordo, 1989, p. 4). Polanyi (1969) created the term "tacit knowing" for learning that occurs in the body. Having rejected the essentialist view of woman as being defined by her body, feminist and critical scholars have recently called for an investigation of the body as a site of (and means of accessing) knowledge (Chodorow, 1989, 1995; Fay, 1987; Flax, 1990; Henderson, 1992; hooks & West, 1991). Several feminist scholars have called for a psychoanalytic exploration of the ways in which the body interprets social and psychological experiences and the ways in which the mind interprets the experiences of the body (Chodorow, 1989; Flax, 1990; hooks & West, 1991). Within that context, I have suggested that a feminist nursing perspective calls for a new definition of gender identity that acknowledges the tacit, bodily knowing of self as a gendered and sexual being (Henderson, 1992).

More specifically, Fay (1987) offers an example of how bodily knowing is transmitted and suggests methods of consciousness-raising that may access that knowing. These methods may be of particular value to nurses engaged in emancipatory action, as we are more likely to deal with bodies and may be more aware of the interconnections of the body-mind than others doing consciousness-raising practice. Fay posits that beliefs are "imprinted in the muscles, organs, nerves, and skeletons" and uses the examples of infants learning from the touch and handling of their parents and children learning from the physical environment of schools (p. 152). He suggests such bodywork techniques as rolfing and yoga as possible emancipatory actions.

An example of consciousness-raising occurring through the body occurred for me during my involvement with the women's program. I participated in a marathon, day-long women's group that I had envisioned as involving hours of talk therapy. What took place was quite different from what I had expected. The day consisted of, among other things, singing together, eating together, doing yoga, teaching and learning a dance step called the hustle, doing role plays, and having a beauty shop. Each of these events involved consciousness-raising and the transmission of knowledge in ways that were more than verbal and cognitive. I want to focus here on the beauty shop experience.

The beauty shop was set up after lunch, complete with straight combs, shampoo, and gels. Most of the women were African American, but there were a number of European American women there. Anyone who wanted could have her hair cut, washed, set, and styled. Two staff members and three residents were quite adept at styling hair, and one staff member had been a professional haircutter in the past, so she did all the cuts. Several of the rest of us did the shampooing. I washed women's hair in a tiny sink. Many different kinds of hair—straight, curly, nappy, kinky—waited to be gelled, finger waved, straightened. What did I learn that day? I learned about straight combs, about heat applied to hair to straighten, about finger waves, about hair that has a texture and feel very different from mine. Some of this I learned through my fingers as I washed other women's hair and helped in the settings. I became aware of my assumptions about black people's hair, which I had thought was tough, bristly, wiry (read, unpleasant). I was surprised at how soft and pleasing it was to touch. On a deep level, I felt myself cross a skin boundary as I touched black women. I had touched black women before, but the intimacy of washing someone's hair allowed me to be present to the experience in a way I had not been before. I felt my racism in my body, rather than through my intellect, a vastly different experience. At the same time, on an intellectual level, I confronted my more feminist political assumption that straightening hair is a regressive thing to do. As I watched the skill with which the women crafted finger waves and the pleasure women experienced in owning them, I had to suspend my critique while I joined in the admiration.

Reflecting on that experience from this moment 2 years later, I confess to some trepidation about revealing my own lack of consciousness about racism. Producing thoughts in text is like applying a fixative, making something hard and material in time and space. In reality, my glimpse into my sense of separation from black women was a fragile and momentary awakening that has continued to have an impact in my life. That awareness was one of many that have led to changes in my own attitudes and behavior. Becoming aware of unconscious and long-held assumptions is the first step in changing those assumptions and the behaviors associated with them. That awareness and change have ultimately been liberating for me, creating more openness and honesty in my relationships with other women.

Bodily knowings, knowledge gained through the emotions, knowledge based on experience, and knowledge that is located within a particular context are valid in feminist consciousness-raising. These sources/types of knowledge challenge and expand our previous understandings of knowledge as being universal, rational, cognitive, and objective. As nurses, we can both benefit from and contribute to the exploration of this expanded understanding.

CONSCIOUSNESS-RAISING WITHIN A FEMINIST NURSING PERSPECTIVE

Within a feminist nursing perspective, consciousness-raising involves an engagement by nurses with others in a mutual process of enlightenment, empowerment, and emancipation. During this engagement, knowledge that is embodied, emotional, contextual, and experiential is produced. Knowledge production is part of the healing process of emancipation (Henderson, 1995b). Although she uses the term *expanding consciousness* rather than *consciousness-raising,* Margaret Newman (1986) provides a language that explains this process. Newman defines consciousness as the informational capacity of the human being—it is not only a mental process, but exists in all of the bodily systems. Genetic coding, the endocrine system, and the immune system are all examples of information-carrying systems within the human body that contribute to the consciousness of the system. The process of health, which contains both illness and wellness, is the process of expanding consciousness.

While not limiting consciousness to mental processes, Newman identifies the experience of insight as crucial to expanded levels of consciousness in humans. With this insight, people are able to gain an understanding of the patterns that make up who they are. Health in humans is the process of coming to understand the patterns of one's relationship with the environment through the insights gained by recognizing those patterns. By understanding his or her pattern, a person can achieve more evolved levels of consciousness.

Newman's explanations are consistent with a feminist perspective of consciousness-raising as an emancipatory process (Henderson, 1995b). Health is a process of emancipation, of becoming more fully human via expanded consciousness. At the same time, a feminist nursing view of health does not allow the emphasis to rest solely on the individual, but reinforces the interrelationship of the personal and the political. Empowerment implies not just action or change for personal health, but social action to redress power imbalances that are impediments to health.

Consciousness-raising is a powerful tool for personal and political awakening and can be a valuable feminist nursing action. In this chapter, I have advocated the reconsideration of this method within the critique of earlier formulations of feminist and critical theories out of which the concept of consciousness-raising developed. Postmodern feminists and feminists of color have helped us to see the importance of considering our own location within the group and the differences of power and privilege among group members based on the social construction of identities and varying levels of knowledge and experience. Feminist and nursing theorists have expanded our concept of what constitutes valid knowledge and its sources. Based on these insights, I want to close with some reflections on (not prescriptions for) the future of consciousness-raising as a feminist nursing action, what Weiler (1994) calls "a more complex realization of the Freirean vision of a collective conscientization" (p. 35).

This new vision asks us to recognize that consciousness-raising must take place in coalitions of people with varying identities. We are called on, therefore, to be more self-reflective in our work and in our writing about our work as feminist nurses. We need to situate ourselves within a social and historical context, acknowledge our multiple identities and our places of power and privilege, and talk about the raising of our own consciousnesses, and not just those of the group members with whom we engage. Power differences that are located within the group need to be articulated and addressed, including those that occur because we are nurses, professionals, and getting paid for the work.

Conflicts within consciousness-raising groups can be openly encountered and explored as potential sources of strength and greater growth. We also need to admit and deal with the pain and loss that occurs in consciousness-raising.

Remembering that consciousness-raising is a political act, not just a personal one, will continue to be a challenge for feminists and feminist nurses. Consciousness-raising is not therapy, nor is it a component of therapy. Consciousness-raising must include an integration of social and individual change.

As feminist nurses, we are expanding our understanding of what constitutes knowledge. Acknowledging the role of the emotions in knowledge production is one step. Exploring the development of knowing in the body is another, one that I think is particularly exciting for nurses who work with the body and have conceptualized the integration of the body-mind. There is great potential in looking beyond dialogue to other forms of human interactions as methods of consciousness-raising.

In consciousness-raising, we ask those with whom we engage to open their minds, to challenge their long-held assumptions, to break free of their ideological and material fetters, to forge emancipatory visions out of old constraints, and to bring those visions to fruition in their lives and in society. My hope for our future as feminist nursing practitioners is that we acknowledge the grandiosity of that goal, confront the real-life ambiguities and limitations of the endeavor, and continue to engage in the struggle, redefining consciousness-raising as our own consciousnesses are raised.

REFERENCES

Chodorow, N. (1989). *Feminism and psychoanalytic theory.* New Haven, CT: Yale University Press.

Chodorow, N. (1995). Gender as a personal and cultural construction. *Signs, 20,* 516-544.

Collins, P. H. (1990). *Black feminist thought: Knowledge, consciousness and the politics of empowerment.* New York: Routledge.

Fay, B. (1987). *Critical social science: Liberation and its limits.* Ithaca, NY: Cornell University Press.

Fisher, B. (1987). The heart has its reasons: Feeling, thinking and community building in feminist education. *Women's Studies Quarterly, 15*(3/4), 40-58.

Flax, J. (1990). *Thinking fragments: Psychoanalysis, feminism, and postmodernism in the contemporary West.* Berkeley: University of California Press.

Fonow, M. M., & Cook, J. A. (1991). *Beyond methodology: Feminist scholarship as lived research.* Bloomington: Indiana University Press.

Frankenberg, R. (1993). *White women, race matters: The social construction of whiteness.* Minneapolis: University of Minnesota Press.

Freire, P. (1990). *Pedagogy of the oppressed* (M. Ramos, Trans.). New York: Continuum. (Original work published 1970)

Gibson, C. (1991). A concept analysis of empowerment. *Journal of Advanced Nursing, 16,* 354-361.

Hagedorn, S. (1995). The politics of caring: The role of activism in primary care. *Advances in Nursing Science, 17*(4), 1-11.

Henderson, D. (1992). Is woman born or made? Female gender identity and women's health. In J. Thompson, D. Allen, & L. Rodrigues-Fisher (Eds.), *Critique and freedom: Working papers in politics of nursing* (pp. 117-128). New York: National League for Nursing.

Henderson, D. (1995a). Consciousness-raising in participatory research: Method and methodology for emancipatory nursing inquiry. *Advances in Nursing Science, 17*(3), 58-69.

Henderson, D. (1995b). Feminist nursing participatory research with black and white women in drug treatment. *Dissertations Abstracts International, 55*(09).

hooks, b. (1992, July/August). Out of the academy and into the streets. *Ms., 3,* 80-82.

hooks, b., & West, C. (1991). *Breaking bread.* Boston: South End.

Jaggar, A., & Bordo, S. (Eds.). (1989). *Gender, body, knowledge: Feminist reconstructions of being and knowing.* New Brunswick, NJ: Rutgers University Press.

Kendall, J. (1992). Fighting back: Promoting emancipatory nursing actions. *Advances in Nursing Science, 15*(2), 1-15.

Kieffer, C. (1984). Citizen empowerment: A developmental perspective. In J. Rappaport, C. Swift, & R. Hess (Eds.), *Studies in empowerment: Toward understanding and action.* New York: Haworth.

Lather, P. (1991). *Getting smart: feminist research and pedagogy with/in the postmodern.* New York: Routledge.

MacKinnon, C. (1989). *Toward a feminist theory of state.* Cambridge, MA: Harvard University Press.

Moccia, P. (1988). At the fault line: Social activism and caring. *Nursing Outlook, 36,* 30-33.

Narayan, U. (1989). The project of feminist epistemology: Perspectives from a non-Western feminist. In A. Jaggar & S. Bordo (Eds.), *Gender, body, knowledge: Feminist reconstructions of being and knowing* (pp. 256-269). New Brunswick, NJ: Rutgers University Press.

Newman, M. (1986). *Health as expanding consciousness.* St. Louis, MO: C. V. Mosby.

Polanyi, M. (1969). *Knowing and being.* Chicago: University of Chicago Press.

Pratt, M. (1984). Identity: Skin, blood, heart. In E. Bulkin, M. Pratt, & B. Smith (Eds.), *Yours in struggle: Three feminist perspectives on anti-Semitism and racism* (pp. 11-63). Ithaca, NY: Firebrand.

Reagon, B. (1983). Coalition politics: Turning the century. In B. Smith (Ed.), *Home girls: A black feminist anthology* (pp. 356-368). New York: Kitchen Table.

Rosenthal, N. (1984). Consciousness-raising: From revolution to re-evaluation. *Psychology of Women Quarterly, 8,* 309-326.

Sampselle, C. (1991). The role of nursing in preventing violence against women. *Journal of Obstetric, Gynecological and Neonatal Nursing, 20,* 481-487.

Sieng, S., & Thompson, J. (1992). Traces of Khmer women's imaginary: Finding our way in the West. *Women and Therapy, 13,* 129-139.

Stevens, P., & Hall, J. (1992). Applying critical theories to nursing in communities. *Public Health Nursing, 9,* 2-9.

Thompson, J. (1991). Exploring gender and culture with Khmer refugee women: Reflections on participatory feminist research. *Advances in Nursing Science, 13*(3), 30-48.

Weiler, K. (1994). Freire and a feminist pedagogy of difference. In P. McLaren & C. Lankshear (Eds.), *Politics of liberation: Paths from Freire* (pp. 12-39). London: Routledge.

Wheeler, C., & Chinn, P. (1991). *Peace and power: A handbook of feminist process.* New York: National League for Nursing.

Woods, N. (1995). Frameworks for nursing practice with women. In C. Ingram-Fogle & N. Woods (Eds.), *Women's health care: A comprehensive handbook* (pp. 125-140). Thousand Oaks, CA: Sage.

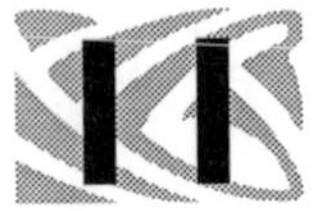

The Revolution Never Ends

Challenges of Praxis for Nursing Education

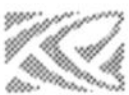

COLLEEN VARCOE

"You still use the word *noncompliance.* You're still calling me a 'patient,' a 'diabetic.' You're still teaching nurses to tell me what my goals are!" Helene responds to my oppressive practices as an educator with gentle persistence, grim determination, a forbearing sort of anger. Helene is intelligent, strong, passionate, a colleague who draws on her experiences with diabetes, cardiac disease, renal failure, and the health care system to advise and teach me. But Helene could never be defined by these experiences.

As a nursing educator for the past 15 or so years, I have engaged in a journey of personal and professional development much like the one so reflectively and eloquently described by Em Bevis (1993). I have struggled to cast off the shackles of behaviorism and Tylerism, and to resist the seductive lure of power over students. I have considered myself progressive, enlightened by study of adult education and sustained by visionary nurse educators. But people like Helene keep me from being too self-satisfied, too self-congratulatory, and from thinking I have come to a place of rest.

Nursing education is moving away from its traditional roots, toward liberatory, transformative, or emancipatory curricula in a movement that has been termed the curriculum revolution. Curriculum is evolving from content applied in practice to curriculum as praxis. To this point, visionary nurse educators have concentrated on the emancipation of the student-teacher relationship and the reform of educational contexts. In this chapter, I will propose that we build on the advances of the past decade by extending our focus and emancipatory philosophy beyond the student-teacher relationship to the client and the nurse-client relationship and by critically analyzing what constitutes content within a curriculum-as-praxis. I will suggest that these advances require placing the client at the center of the curriculum. Such a shift is predicated on ideas regarding the nature of praxis, who has truth and knowledge, and the legitimate sites of nursing knowledge production.

PREMISES OF PRAXIS

The use of the term *praxis* in nursing ranges from the liberal to the radical sense of the concept. Liberal apolitical notions of praxis are confined to the ideas of reflection on one's own practice and consideration of the dialectic relationship between reflection and action, theory, and practice. Praxis in its more radical sense—or, in Freire's (1970/1993) terms, "revolutionary praxis"—encompasses reflection on the world and action toward emancipatory purpose. Ford and Profetto-McGrath (1994) contend that there are "two moments to critical reflection. One relates to a critical examination of one's own practice. The other relates to the need for a critical understanding of the way the system works to maintain the status quo" (p. 343). Grundy (1987) argues that action in praxis transforms, rather than maintains, the status quo, changing "both the world and our understanding of that world" (p. 113). Action in revolutionary praxis is also focused both on oneself and on the world and, because praxis implies an emancipatory purpose, both reflection and action are directed toward emancipation.

I believe that revolutionary praxis is fundamental to the curriculum revolution in nursing. Freire (1970/1993) argues that there is a "praxis of the dominant elites," but contends that revolutionary praxis is antithetical to, and must stand in opposition to, a praxis (theory and practice, reflection and action) of domination. He argues that education can be a tool of liberation or a weapon of oppression. Reflection and action without the goal of emancipation may be mere musing upon and maintenance of the status quo. And education without revolutionary praxis is an instrument of oppression.

Central to liberatory pedagogy is the question of who is being emancipated or empowered, and by whom. Gore (1992) argues that in education there are discourses of empowerment that are conservative (equating empowerment with professionalization) or liberal (focusing on empowerment of individual students and teachers and on power relations *within* the classroom), and critical or feminist discourses concerned with power relations at the social and collective level that are more overtly political. Thus in these three discourses, reflection and action focus on the individual student, the student-teacher relationship, and the wider social context, respectively.

Fundamental to the very idea of education is the idea that someone (usually the teacher) has more knowledge and power than someone else (the student), making education an essentially paternalistic project (Ellsworth, 1989). In critical and feminist pedagogy, the teacher is usually cast as the agent of empowerment and the student as the object, with the student constructed as oppressed. However, several authors within this discourse caution against empowerment or liberation as guises for paternalism. Freire (1970/1993) argues that one cannot validly carry out transformation *for* the oppressed, only *with* the oppressed. Analyzing empowerment in education, Gore (1992) criticizes thinking of power as a commodity and as oppositional to oppression, and charges that positioning the educator as an agent of empowerment sets up "them" (who are oppressed) and "us" who have power. She contends that educators with emancipatory intent would do better to focus on assisting others to exercise their own power, rather than on "sharing" power. This view is similar to arguments that the idea of "giving voice" is oppositional and paternalistic and should be replaced with the idea of making space for others to speak (e.g., Alcoff, 1992; Ellsworth, 1989).

These arguments are related to the issue of who has truth and knowledge. Freire's stance is based on the idea that all people are subjects with their own agency, capable of reflection and action in their own right. Ellsworth (1989) argues against the teacher as central on the basis that, as all knowledge is partial and often contradictory and as social positions are multiple and often oppositional, the teacher cannot know students' oppression or define what is emancipatory. "Unity" is not "sameness," the teacher will never access all knowledge, and a pooling of all available partial knowledges is essential. Holding the teacher as central maintains the teacher as predominant; holding the student-teacher relationship as central implies it is the primary site of knowledge creation.

As yet, radical philosophies of education and critical pedagogical theories fail to provide meaningful direction regarding how to analyze or redress the institutional power imbalances between students and teachers (Ellsworth, 1989). Gore (1992) notes:

> In the attempt not to impose an agenda on others, critical pedagogy discourses have opted instead for rather abstract theories of empowerment. And yet, they have imposed on teachers the requirement to do the work of empowering, . . . without providing much in the way of tangible guidance for that work. (p. 66)

Gore argues that the guidance she calls for must come from closer attention to the contexts in which empowerment is to occur. Thus to analyze praxis in nursing, we must examine the context of nursing education to consider the focus of reflection and action, to ask who is being empowered by whom, to identify who has knowledge and truth, and to determine where knowledge is produced.

PRAXIS IN NURSING EDUCATION

Historically, nursing education has been extremely conservative, and nurses have only recently drawn from radical philosophies of education and adult education to incorporate theories, strategies, and concepts such as praxis. In nursing the increasing popularity of the term *praxis* has coincided with what has been called the curriculum revolution. Educators such as Bevis, Watson, Diekelmann, and Tanner have challenged the traditions of nursing education and have called for the revolutionizing of student-teacher relationships. Many have responded and are now engaged in the challenges of praxis.

The Focus of Reflection and Action

In nursing's curriculum revolution, the primary focus of reflection and action has been on student-teacher interactions within the teaching-learning context. Reflection on one's own practice (especially the educator's) has been emphasized; actions have been taken by educators to challenge and transform the educational context and status quo.

Although social responsibility is identified as a central theme of the curriculum revolution (Tanner, 1990b), attention to the practice context has been marginal. Munhall (1988) has suggested processes for confronting injustice and inequalities arising from the health care system and society in nursing's shift from a military metaphor to a metaphor of advocacy, but most attention in nursing education has remained on the educational process itself. Similarly, Bevis and Watson (1989) have called for moves away from oppressive educational *and* practice structures, but their interest concerns predominantly educational structures. With a few exceptions, such as Spence (1994), who has called for explicit attention to health care settings and nursing organizations, practice structures have received little analysis in nursing education literature. Even when changes to the practice context are advocated, benefits are usually discussed in terms of students (e.g., Bevis, 1989; McLeod & Farrell, 1994). Although nurses call for curriculum driven by the *realities* of practice, they have paid scant attention to transforming those realities and less attention to transforming the client's world within the nursing practice context.

The Focus of Empowerment

Empowerment of students has been the initial concern of the curriculum revolution in nursing, and the primary agent of empowerment has usually been the teacher. There is, however, growing acknowledgment of the student as an active agent in the educational process. With emphasis on the educational context, empowerment of the client has not been central, and the agency of clients, and students in relationship with clients, has not been fundamental to educational analyses. As in other areas of critical pedagogy, practical ways to reformulate these power relationships require further development.

It is important to note that preoccupation with the empowerment of nurses and inattention to practice structures are not confined to the educational literature. Most nursing literature concerned with empowerment, analyses of power, and praxis is focused on nurses' power, powerlessness, oppressed group behavior, and potential for empowerment. The client has been marginalized in most of such discussions, and, as Spence (1994) notes, the hegemonic influences of institutions are not addressed.

The Site of Knowledge Production

The student-teacher relationship has been seen as the primary site of knowledge production in recent nursing educational theory. In Bevis and Watson's (1989) highly influential text, curriculum is defined as "the interactions and transactions that occur between and among students and teachers with the intent that learning occur" (p. 5). This definition highlights central assumptions of nursing's curriculum revolution: The student (as well as the teacher) has truth and knowledge, and interaction between students is a site of knowledge production. Alternative definitions, such as those offered by Diekelmann (1988) and Nelms (1991), remain concerned primarily with the student-teacher relationship as the site of knowledge production. There is recognition that students learn from their experiences with clients; however, the client is not usually conceptualized as an active agent in that learning or as a source of truth and knowledge.

To this point in nursing's curriculum revolution, significant emphasis has been placed on reforming student-teacher relationships and the educational context, and on empowering students as active partners in the learning relationship. However, when the educational context is privileged over the practice context, and emancipatory efforts focus on the student, the teacher-as-nurse and student-as-nurse are obscured and the nurse-client relationship as a site of oppression is not addressed. Revolutionary praxis draws attention beyond the educational context to the wider context of nursing, that is, to the practice context. Locating praxis for nursing education within practice extends the focus of reflection beyond the student-teacher relationship to the nurse-client relationship, and challenges not just the structures that maintain the status quo of education, but those that maintain the status quo of the context of health and health care. Emancipatory goals then encompass the client as well as the nurse. If empowerment is theorized as *doing with,* as moving over to make space for others to exercise their power, and if the client is conceptualized as having truth, knowledge, and agency, then there is a basis for renegotiating the role of the client in nursing education.

THE PATIENT IS PALE

The patient is largely absent from writings on educational reform in nursing, and the patient's world is at a distance from the educational context. Despite the leadership of nurse educators who draw attention to the oppression of clients (e.g., Tanner, 1990a), there is little discussion in the nursing education literature of the oppression of people with illness and disabilities, of power relationships in practice settings, or of the nurse-patient relationship as a site of oppression. In fact, Watson (1989) calls for a "pedagogy of the non-oppressed" for nursing (p. 43). Even with moves to phenomenological approaches, where "new possibilities for curriculum and instruction will emerge that are grounded in the day to day experiences of clinicians, students, and teachers" (Diekelmann, 1990, p. 301), the client is absent, unless perhaps as an implicit object of others' experiences.

As in theoretical curriculum literature, in clinical education the patient role is usually quite passive. Chopoorian (1990) argues that "patients . . . are mostly invisible to faculty, their clinical and life problems take a secondary place to the educational process" (p. 23). In my own practice I see that patients are "used" as "experiences" for students. In the intensive care unit, it is rare for anyone to consider whether the patient, even when conscious, is willing to be cared for by a student. In the renal unit, patient cooperation is obtained, but the person is often objectified and essentialized. Helene says, "I hate it when they talk over me like I'm not there. 'How much fluid is she taking off?' they say."

I am interested in why we speak of the emancipation of students without speaking of emancipation of clients. Do we see ourselves as educators, but not as clinicians? Do we see our students as only students, not as practitioners? Do we see education as an end in itself, and have no clear view of the uses to which students will put the knowledge they acquire? Do we think that whereas one philosophy is necessary for education, another is sufficient for practice? Why do we seek to rid ourselves of oppressive behavior toward students yet fail to challenge our behavior toward clients and the same in students? Why, despite growing critical scholarship in nursing focused on oppression of clients, is marginal attention given to these issues in the nursing education literature? Is the theory-practice gap in nursing so wide that these issues have not been considered? Or do educators simply begin in the best place for reflection and action: their own practice?

This is not to say that the client has not been considered at all. Caring is a core value of nursing's curriculum revolution (Tanner, 1990a, 1990b) and serves as the foundation for the nurse-patient relationship. For example, Bevis and Watson (1989) state that nursing's unique societal mission is "to care for the vulnerable and to provide caring services in prevention, cure and maintenance" (p. 350).

The concept of caring is problematic, owing to lack of definition and multiple definitions and interpretations (see Morse, Bottorff, Neander, & Solberg, 1991; Phillips, 1993; Thomas, 1993), although, as Munhall (1988) observes, the concept of caring is itself undergoing a transformation. "Caring" has had limited analysis in nursing education (Paterson & Crawford, 1994) and is particularly problematic within a liberatory curriculum because educators pay limited attention to the relationship between caring and praxis. Paterson and Crawford (1994) contend that, in nursing education, caring has generally been seen as a precursor to empowerment. Bevis and Watson (1989) speak of a "praxis of caring," where "theory and practice live together, each informing the other" (p. 56). However, they do not discuss the relationship between this praxis of caring and emancipation or empowerment, which are definitional of revolutionary praxis.

Caring is also seen as essential to education in dealing with power imbalances in health care institutions and the challenge of preparing nurses for practice in institutions that do not necessarily serve the health care needs of people (Tanner, 1990a; Watson, 1989). Bevis and Watson (1989) contend that a praxis of caring is "first applied (in educational settings) and later translated from pedagogical practices into the clinical world of nursing practice" (p. 56). However, direction for accomplishing this translation to practice and the prerequisite analysis of practice structures are absent in nursing education.

Analyses of caring undertaken from critical and feminist perspectives have questioned the compatibility of caring and empowerment, and have concluded that an ethic of care is at best only partially sufficient for practice (e.g. Houston, 1990; Malin & Teasdale, 1991; Olsen, 1993). Houston (1990) charges that the relational ontology of an ethic of caring makes caring dangerous, as it can abet exploitation. Ellsworth (1989) maintains that in education, code words such as *critical* and *social change* have effectively masked the political agenda of liberatory educators, rendering the critical education movement invisible and bereft of a "clear articulation of the need for its existence, goals, risks or potentials" (p. 300). Similarly in nursing education, terms such as *caring* may have depoliticized the curriculum "revolution" by making both students and clients the objects of caring rather than agents of change. There is a danger that the use of the concept of caring, without analysis of its relationship to empowerment and praxis, may preclude the extension of a liberatory philosophy to the client of nursing. The client may be conceptualized as an object of caring, as the recipient of care, as the source of "problems" for caring nurses to solve. With no explicit establishment of the agency of the client, clients may be conceptualized as the powerless "them" in contrast to "us" and essentialized to the patient role. Caring may mask the power relations between nurses and clients, leaving the potential for paternalism unconsidered. The praxis of caring may become a praxis of domination.

The incongruence of a liberatory philosophy for student-teacher relationships and paternalistic philosophy for nurse-patient relationships cannot be resolved with a simple shift from empowering students to empowering patients, both of which are predicated on unequal power relations. Rather, a complex understanding of the nature of empowerment, the focus of reflection and action, and the sites of knowledge production must undergird curricular reconstruction. If praxis is to underlie nursing curriculum, then emancipation of clients and the nurse-client relationship must be foremost, and the client must be moved to the center of the curriculum in a meaningful manner.

There has been little interchange between critical scholarship in nursing and trends toward a critical pedagogy in nursing education. Analysis of the social context of health and health care, transformation of the client's world, and client empowerment have been central to critical scholarship in nursing during the past decade. Feminist theory, critical social theory, and postmodern and poststructuralist approaches have been used to initiate a growing critical tradition in nursing. Reconceptualization of the client of nursing, the environment, and the nurse-client relationship, and attention to the social determinants of health and all forms of oppression are but a few of the domains advanced by critical scholars. These ideas provide a resource for moving beyond liberal notions of praxis and for examining the content and process of nursing education.

THE CONTENT IS NEBULOUS

Overthrowing the tyranny of content has been a central struggle for educators invested in the "new paradigm" of nursing curriculum. Allen (1990b) has called for nursing education to cast off the tyranny of content by moving toward process, and, as Moccia (1990b) has remarked, "process has become substance" (p. 309). The need to have new educational processes has overshadowed the need for analysis of the impact of emancipatory intent on content. With the focus predominantly on the student-teacher relationship, curriculum revisions profoundly alter the process of education, but either abandon the content to be defined through the process or leave the content unexamined. Perhaps now we have revised process sufficiently to be ready to rethink content.

Content needs to be addressed. Grundy (1987) points out that curriculum-as-praxis does not mean that the teacher does not have a role in deciding the content and that negotiated curriculum does not mean "anything goes" (p. 122). Nursing educators recognize that content is an important issue (e.g., Bevis & Watson, 1989; Chopoorian, 1990; Ford & Profetto-McGrath, 1994), but as yet concrete direction is limited.

From the late 1960s to the mid-1980s, content in nursing was increasingly derived from nursing models. Pleas for theoretical pluralism and dissatisfaction with nursing models (or perhaps dissatisfaction with tyrannical and obsessive implementation of models) displaced formal nursing models as a source of content. Furthermore, some critics argue that most nursing theories are irrelevant and acontextual, and that they perpetuate patriarchal ideologies of society (e.g., Lutjens & Horan, 1992; Wilson-Thomas, 1995), suggesting incompatibility between nursing models and liberatory curricula. However, nurse educators offer few alternative approaches to determining content.

If nursing models (which attempt to define, among other things, the unique role of nursing, the client of nursing, and the goal of nursing) are not to guide curriculum, then how is content to be determined in a manner congruent with a liberatory curriculum that extends to the client of nursing? Although Bevis and Watson (1989) argue for the centrality of patient experiences to nursing, they do not include such experiences among their suggested sources of content, and there has been little subsequent attention to content in the literature. Phenomenological approaches in education remain centered on the experiences of students, teachers, and nurses (e.g. Diekelmann, 1995; Nehls, 1995), with little direct attention to the lived experience of clients.

Before turning to the issue of what content should be addressed within curriculum as praxis, I think it is important to acknowledge that not all interests in nursing curricula are directly concerned with emancipation. Using Habermas's distinctions among technical, practical, and emancipatory interests, Allen (1990a) emphasizes the importance of identifying and debating which interest is operating. I am specifically concerned here with the implications for content arising from emancipatory interests.

CURRICULUM CONTENT FOR PRAXIS

I propose that content in curriculum-as-praxis arises directly from what is meant by *praxis*. If praxis in nursing education is concerned with reflection and action on the self and the world, and if, as I have argued, the world of nursing is concerned with the client and the environment as it affects health, then these are the sources of content. If praxis is also concerned with emancipation, then the sites of oppression, the nature of power, and the processes of empowerment are additional sources of content.

The Client as a Source of Content

If we are to have curriculum that aims to be liberatory for clients, nurse educators must make room for clients to exercise their power within that curriculum. The determination of what is important to teach nurses about clients must therefore come from clients themselves. Although individual client experiences may be used as sources of content in phenomenological approaches in the clinical setting, such learning may be limited to the immediate experiences of the individual client and student. This approach may foster an understanding of the unique experiences of individuals, but it does not foster an understanding of aggregates of experience, of the commonalities of experience that are essential to guide nursing practice. Further, analysis at the level of individual students and clients may be lost in the immediacy of the experience and may fail to take into account the larger social structures in which the experiences are embedded.

Attending to aggregates of client experience as a source of content can be achieved in at least two ways: first, by using both qualitative and quantitative research derived directly from the experience of clients, and second, through curriculum development processes in which clients determine content. The very presence of client representatives at the curriculum table changes awareness and language. Discussion can no longer proceed in terms of "us" and "them." The perspective of the recipient of care can explode and expand our ideas regarding who the client is, what the goal of nursing is, why the client needs nursing, and what constitutes competence, and can lead to client-oriented content, establish a basis for client-focused practice, and model empowerment in a nonpaternalistic manner.

For example, choice of treatment modality is critical to people with renal disease. In revising a nephrology nursing program, clients expanded our understanding of the complexity of each individual; what client goals are and how they vary in terms of what *empowerment, health,* and *decision making* mean; and what clients need from nursing. Clients explained the decision-making processes they use and taught us that clients change modalities not only for physiological benefit, but also for reasons such as their work and child-care needs, how much social contact with other clients they want, which physician is associated with each treatment type, perceived quality of care in different dialysis units, and the language spoken by most people served by a given unit. Clients illustrated that for decision making they require information, not only about physiological benefits of each type of dialysis, but also about the potential impacts on work, intimate relationships, home environment, costs, travel, and health care, as well as support, encouragement, and advocacy. Viewing the client as a source of knowledge and an active agent suggests that clients are a source of curriculum content at the individual and collective levels, not as passive objects, but as teachers and colearners. Client experiences of, and resources and processes for dealing with, health, illness, and the health care system become content essential to liberatory curricula.

The Environment as a Source of Content

The context of health and health care includes the immediate environments in which health care is delivered and the larger social context. Therefore a major challenge of praxis for nursing education is to extend our targets of reflection and action from educational institutions to the health care system and social systems as they affect health. Rather than the limited move from a curriculum driven by content to a curriculum driven by "the realities of practice," which assumes that the realities of practice are givens, the liberatory curriculum seeks to transform the environment of health and health care.

Attention to the environment has been clearly demanded by authors of the curriculum revolution. In 1989, Watson argued that it was past time for nursing to look at the structural problems in the health care system, and in 1990, Moccia claimed that the reconceptualized environment had emerged as a central theme of the revolution.

Chopoorian (1990) provides direction for deriving content from the environment by identifying two central realities with which the nursing profession needs to contend. First, she asserts that nurses are unable to provide high-quality care in the health care institutions in which they practice, suggesting that nurses must study the contexts of care and the constraints to quality nursing care as well as acquire the skills to overcome those constraints. Second, she stresses that "the nature of health problems today are characterized as being produced by society" (p. 33). She argues that preparing nurses for roles that deal with individual psychological responses to problems, rather than preparing nurses to deal with root causes of health problems, such as stress, crisis, poverty, and malnutrition, actually increases individual problems. Chopoorian clearly suggests content emphasis on the social causes of health problems and on skills to fulfill roles that deal with those causes. This orientation is echoed by Ford and Profetto-McGrath (1994), who argue for attention in nursing education to the "larger socio-political, historical and economic contexts so as to address the fundamental power relationships" (p. 343).

Imagining future graduates of liberatory curricula, Moccia (1990b) says that such nurses will

> expose the layers and layers of patriarchal obfuscation to see the relationship between public policies and private lives; [and] . . . will be found in those activities where definitions of health and health care are being challenged . . . in the politics of challenging the ideology of the health care system and the structure and function of the delivery system. (p. 310)

In this vision lies clear direction for content. Nurses must learn public policy, the structure of health care, and the ways systems operate to define health and health care. The structure of the health care system and society, and the impacts of both on health and health care, becomes essential content for liberatory curricula.

Sites of Oppression as a Source of Content

Liberatory curricula must, by definition, be concerned with oppression. If we are to extend emancipatory intent to our relationships with clients, we must also extend our understanding of oppression beyond the student-teacher relationship. Bevis (1993) critiques the interrelationships between educational structures and the position of nurse educators, saying that "oppression stems from a need to maintain the status quo; most times it is designed to keep those of power and privilege in positions of power and privilege" (p. 102). This understanding can be applied directly to clients, beginning self-reflectively with educator-client and nurse-client relationships as sites of oppression.

Oppression provides an essential source of content. Feminist writers have drawn attention to gender as a site of oppression, and from a feminist perspective nurse educators have argued for particular content. For example, Boughn and Wang (1995) argue for the inclusion of health-related concerns of women's everyday lives that are devalued or ignored in traditional curricula. However, gender is only one site of oppression that is relevant to health care. Race, class, age, sexual orientation, and disability are all sites of oppression that have significant relevance to health and nursing practice. The sites and nature of oppression, the way in which social structures operate, and the nature of power are essential content for liberatory curricula. And with the study of oppression must come the study of resistance and empowerment.

The Processes of Empowerment as a Source of Content

If liberatory curricula focus reflection and action on the structures that maintain the status quo both within the health care system and in the social context of health and health care, then strategies for reflection and action in those spheres become essential to the content of those curricula. Content must include theories useful for the analysis of social structure and strategies for transformation of structures. For example, in teaching client education, I use Mezirow's theory of transformative learning (Cranton, 1994).

Authors such as Grundy (1987) argue that critical social theory is essential to praxis. Wilson-Thomas (1995) says that "critical social theory can assist nurses in analyzing knowledge that is generated from androcentric ideology so that health can be promoted and maintained from a caring, contextual and humanistic perspective" (p. 573). The challenge of praxis is to empower clients, not only students. Thus content must include the nature of empowerment and ways of nursing without dominating.

Curriculum Process for Praxis

Grundy (1987) asserts that in curriculum-as-praxis, the question of the nature of curriculum content cannot be answered apart from questions related to the power of the various participants to determine the content. Although the role of the teacher in nursing education has been critiqued, when the teacher remains at the center of liberatory activities, a transmission-of-knowledge model of education is still assumed, the student is constructed as oppressed (Ellsworth, 1989), and the unequal power relations between student and teacher are unchallenged. In nursing, this focus privileges the student-teacher relationship as the primary site of learning and thus devalues the nurse-client relationship. When Ellsworth (1989), Lather (1991), and others challenge liberatory pedagogies by asking, Who is doing the liberating? they are asking how efforts to liberate perpetuate the relations of dominance and critiquing the ways in which critical educators have failed to come to terms with their positions of power. In nursing these issues need to be addressed in relationship to clients and clinical nurses as well as to students.

Lather (1991) argues that "a central question in rethinking the role of teachers with liberatory intentions" is how we can "position ourselves less as masters of truth and justice and more as creators of a space where those directly involved can act and speak on their own behalf" (p. 137). She notes that the "best solution I have been able to come up with is to position the intellectuals as other than the origin of what can be known and done" (p. 138). One way to do this in nursing education is to recognize students as a source of knowledge and action; another way is to recognize that clients are at the center of every nursing action, and are therefore "directly involved" and need space in the curriculum.

The role of students and the student-teacher relationship in nursing have been critically examined, and reforms have been advocated (Bevis & Watson, 1989; Ford & Profetto-McGrath, 1994), resulting, I believe, in significant shifts toward more egalitarian relationships. However, I sense that these shifts have occurred mostly in immediate, one-to-one relationships between students and teachers. What about the student's role in long-range planning of the curriculum? The legitimate curriculum still appears to be the one implicitly or explicitly agreed upon by the faculty. I have found that students make unique contributions to curriculum, especially in critiquing the appropriateness of assignments and levels of reading, keeping student choice in full view, and forcing the enactment of an emancipatory philosophy. Although the student is increasingly recognized as an active agent in education, revolutionary praxis requires extending this role so that students become full partners in all facets of curriculum. Such partnerships can be created through student representation in all curriculum decisions, from macro-level curriculum design decisions to choices and alternatives in individual learning activities.

The client has had little, if any, role in curriculum development in nursing. Paterson and Crawford (1994) note that little consideration has been given to the idea that anyone other than teachers (including clients) can teach nurses about caring. Clearly, curriculum-as-praxis demands partnerships with clients that are significant and meaningful. Clients can be viewed as active agents, as sources of knowledge, as teachers as well as learners. The clients with whom I work contribute to curricula in many ways. A man whose partner was in intensive care and a woman whose daughter has been in a long-term care facility since birth are working on curriculum committees. Many people with various chronic conditions have contributed their definitions of chronic illness to a specific course. Another group of people with varied experiences with health care are working on a video about those experiences. Here the challenge of praxis is to make space for clients who are most likely to be excluded from such processes, the clients we most need to hear.

Changes in the role of the clinical nurse in curriculum have been demanded by nurses such as Chopoorian (1990) and Bevis and Watson (1989). Chopoorian calls for the collapse of structures in education and for clinical nurses and teachers to live in each other's worlds. By this she does not mean that the distinctions between the worlds of education and practice should be blurred, or that differences in these roles should be obscured; rather, she advocates making space for both in the curriculum. Similarly, Bevis and Watson insist that clinical nurses should be valued and treated as equal partners. In practical terms, this means leaving some control over curriculum to clinical nurses, not only in one-to-one relationships with students, but in the design of the overall curriculum. I have redefined my role in curriculum design and course development as one of providing educational expertise to complement the clinical expertise of clinical colleagues, the experiential expertise of client colleagues, and the learner expertise of student colleagues. However, this is not sufficient. If the clinical nurse is viewed as an active agent and source of knowledge, the nature of nursing knowledge and sites of knowledge production are altered. Maeve (1994) challenges nursing to redefine scholarship in a way that accords the bedside nurse the stature and status of scholar. I suggest that this is another challenge of praxis for nursing education.

Redefining the roles of participants in curriculum development redefines the process. Such changes are neither simple nor easy, and two concerns bear comment. First, as Tanner (1990a) notes, the language of heath care institutions objectifies and dehumanizes people who receive care, and such language pervades our practice. Curriculum-as-praxis requires careful attention to language, with vigilance concerning the labeling and essentializing that are characteristic of the language of domination. Second, if faculty are paid for curriculum work and all input is valued, nonfaculty cannot be expected to "contribute" their time. Clearly, institutional support is required for nonfaculty consultants; this can be compared with the trend toward reimbursing research participants.

IMPLICATIONS OF PRAXIS

A radical philosophy of education would seek to transform not only the relationship between teachers and students, but also the relationship between nurses and clients, and ultimately the health care system. Nurse educators have begun to examine critically their philosophies of education, their roles in relationship to students, and their educational designs and strategies. However, it is my belief that only a radical view of praxis will challenge the status quo of nursing in relation to clients and the social structural constraints within which we practice, for nursing education is not an end in itself, but a means to an end that involves the clients of nursing. Unless students are equipped to transform their relationships with clients and the context of practice, "revolutionized" curricula will only create dissonance and distance between education and practice and put graduates at risk. Nurses educated within a philosophy that espouses egalitarianism, critical thinking, and reflective practice but who do not acquire the skills needed to confront injustice in practice may be placed in positions that maximize their moral distress, reality shock, and frustration.

Strategies to bridge the education-practice gap often focus on creating "bicultural graduates" and on making nursing more congruent with a health care system that is oppressive for both nurses and clients. The current climate in nursing and nursing education offers us the opportunity to unite education and practice by transforming the health care system. Chopoorian (1990) claims that "praxis is our common ground, it unifies our roles, and purpose of existence" (p. 24). Reconceptualizing the client as a central partner in curriculum brings the practice context into sharper focus as the target of action and reflection in nursing praxis, unites theory and practice, and guides educational process and content. Sullivan (1995) claims that a revolution in nursing calls for a shift along two axes: a move toward active learning on the part of the student and a move toward client-centered health care. We have made significant progress toward the first; meeting the challenges of praxis for nursing education depends on the second.

REFERENCES

Alcoff, L. (1992). The problem of speaking for others. *Cultural Critique, 4,* 5-31.

Allen, D. G. (1990a). Critical social theory and nursing education. In National League for Nursing (Ed.), *Curriculum revolution: Redefining the student-teacher relationship* (pp. 67-86). New York: National League for Nursing.

Allen, D. G. (1990b). The curriculum revolution: Radical revisioning of nursing education. *Journal of Nursing Education, 29,* 312-316.

Bevis, E. O. (1989). The curriculum consequences: Aftermath of revolution. In National League for Nursing (Ed.), *Curriculum revolution: Reconceptualizing nursing education* (pp. 115-134). New York: National League for Nursing.

Bevis, E. O. (1993). All in all, it was a pretty good funeral. *Journal of Nursing Education, 32*(3), 101-105.

Bevis, E. O., & Watson, J. (1989). *Toward a caring curriculum: A new pedagogy for nursing.* New York: National League for Nursing.

Boughn, S., & Wang, H. (1995). Introducing a feminist perspective to nursing curricula: A quantitative study. *Journal of Nursing Education, 33,* 112-117.

Chopoorian, T. J. (1990). The two worlds of nursing: The one we teach about, the one that is. In National League for Nursing (Ed.), *Curriculum revolution: Redefining the student-teacher relationship* (pp. 21-36). New York: National League for Nursing.

Cranton, P. (1994). *Understanding and promoting transformative learning: A guide for educators of adults.* San Francisco: Jossey-Bass.

Diekelmann, N. (1988). Curriculum revolution: A theoretical and philosophical mandate for change. In National League for Nursing (Ed.), *Curriculum revolution: Mandate for change* (pp. 137-157). New York: National League for Nursing.

Diekelmann, N. (1990). Nursing education: Caring, dialogue, and practice. *Journal of Nursing Education, 29,* 300-305.

Diekelmann, N. (1995). Reawakening thinking: Is traditional pedagogy nearing completion? *Journal of Nursing Education, 34,* 195-196.

Ellsworth, E. (1989). Why doesn't this feel empowering? Working through the repressive myths of critical pedagogy. *Harvard Educational Review, 59,* 297-324.

Ford, J. S., & Profetto-McGrath, J. (1994). A model for critical thinking within the context of curriculum as praxis. *Journal of Nursing Education, 33,* 341-344.

Freire, P. (1993). *Pedagogy of the oppressed* (M. B. Ramos, Trans.). New York: Continuum. (Original work published 1970)

Gore, J. (1992). What we can do for you! What can "we" do for "you"? Struggling over empowerment in critical and feminist pedagogy. In C. Luke & J. Gore (Eds.), *Feminisms and critical pedagogy* (pp. 54-73). London: Routledge.

Grundy, S. (1987). *Curriculum: Product or praxis?* London: Falmer.

Houston, B. (1990). Caring and exploitation. *Hypatia, 5,* 115-119.

Lather, P. (1991). *Getting smart: Feminist research and pedagogy with/in the postmodern.* New York: Routledge.

Lutjens, L., & Horan, M. (1992). Nursing education: An educational imperative. *Journal of Professional Nursing, 8,* 276-281.

Maeve, M. K. (1994). The carrier bag theory of nursing practice. *Advances in Nursing Science, 16*(4), 9-22.

Malin, N., & Teasdale, K. (1991). Caring versus empowerment: Considerations for nursing practice. *Journal of Advanced Nursing, 16,* 657-662.

McLeod, M. L. P., & Farrell, P. (1994). The need for significant reform: A practice driven approach to curriculum. *Journal of Nursing Education, 33,* 208-214.

Moccia, P. (1990a). Foreword. In National League for Nursing (Ed.), *Curriculum revolution: Community building and activism* (pp. vii-x). New York: National League for Nursing.

Moccia, P. (1990b). No Sire, it's a revolution. *Journal of Nursing Education, 29,* 307-311.

Morse, J. M., Bottorff, J., Neander, W., & Solberg, S. (1991). Comparative analysis of conceptualizations and theories of caring. *Image: The Journal of Nursing Scholarship, 23,* 119-126.

Munhall, P. L. (1988). Curriculum revolution: A social mandate for change. In National League for Nursing (Ed.), *Curriculum revolution: Mandate for change* (pp. 217-230). New York: National League for Nursing.

Nehls, N. (1995). Narrative pedagogy: Rethinking nursing education. *Journal of Nursing Education, 34,* 204-210.

Nelms, T. P. (1991). Has the curriculum revolution revolutionized the definition of curriculum? *Journal of Nursing Education, 30,* 5-8.

Olsen, D. P. (1993). Populations vulnerable to the ethics of caring. *Journal of Advanced Nursing, 18,* 1696-1700.

Paterson, B., & Crawford, M. (1994). Caring in nursing education: An analysis. *Journal of Advanced Nursing, 19,* 164-173.

Phillips, P. (1993). A deconstruction of caring. *Journal of Advanced Nursing, 18,* 1554-1558.

Spence, D. G. (1994). The curriculum revolution: Can educational reform take place without a revolution in practice? *Journal of Advanced Nursing, 19,* 187-193.

Sullivan, E. J. (1995). Education: A revolution in the making. *Journal of Professional Nursing, 11,* 137.

Tanner, C. (1990a). Caring as a value in nursing education. *Nursing Outlook, 38,* 70-72.

Tanner, C. (1990b). Reflections on the curriculum revolution. *Journal of Nursing Education 29,* 295-299.

Thomas, C. (1993). De-constructing concepts of care. *Sociology, 27,* 649-669.

Watson, J. (1989). A new paradigm of curriculum development. In E. O. Bevis & J. Watson, *Toward a caring curriculum: A new pedagogy for nursing* (pp. 37-49). New York: National League for Nursing.

Wilson-Thomas, L. (1995). Applying critical social theory in nursing education to bridge the gap between theory, research and practice. *Journal of Advanced Nursing, 21,* 568-575.

PART III

Emancipatory Inquiry

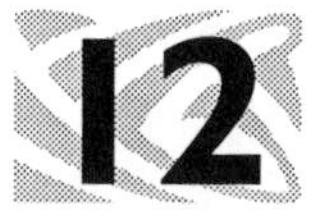

Foundational Thought in the Development of Knowledge for Social Change

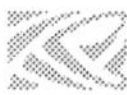

LYNNE E. MAXWELL

Current perspectives on health suggest that persons living in lower socioeconomic groups are at higher risk for disease and disability when compared with those living in higher socioeconomic groups and that these inequalities go beyond medical and behavioral issues to social and political factors (Evans & Stoddart, 1990; Ministry of Supply and Services Canada, 1994; Registered Nurses' Association of British Columbia, 1992). Theories for nursing generally lack direction for nurses to include social activism as part of their practice (Moccia, 1988). Emancipatory nursing is emerging as an important theoretical perspective that challenges nurses to work as social activists to help people overcome social inequalities as a central strategy for enhancing health (Butterfield, 1990).

My purpose in this chapter is to articulate select philosophical foundations for emancipatory nursing. Emancipatory nursing provides direction for nurses to work with the oppressed in such a way that social inequalities influencing health are identified, uncovered, and/or confronted—this in stark contrast to traditional nursing (Butterfield, 1990; Kendall, 1992). Whereas traditional nursing aligns with dominant interests to help people adapt to their oppression, emancipatory nursing aligns with the oppressed to help people take action to change the forces that maintain the status quo (Kendall, 1992; Moccia, 1988). Social change, then, is a central concern of emancipatory nursing. This is no small transformation. Now nursing, once comfortably aligned with dominant social and political groups, is in direct opposition to some of them. To effect the transition from traditional nursing to emancipatory nursing, an understanding of foundational thought in the development of knowledge for social change provides nurses with conceptual material to develop convincing theories to guide practice and research.

I begin the chapter with a brief discussion of emancipatory nursing that identifies the historical roots of nursing science and practice and locates emancipatory nursing within foundational knowledge for social change with reference to the work of Rousseau, Marx, Freire, and Habermas. Rousseau's critical discourse represents an important critique of domination (Luke, 1990). Further, solutions to social inequality proposed by Rousseau are foundational to social and political structures of twentieth-century democratic societies (Baradat, 1994; Luke, 1990). Rousseau's work presages the theoretical work of Marx and the critical social theorists, such as Habermas, whose work is also addressed here (Baradat, 1994). Marx's theories are centrally concerned with social change and introduce the notion of praxis, a key concept in emancipatory nursing. I include discussion of Habermas's theoretical positions here to introduce a critical social theorist whose work is centrally concerned with social change. Freire's perspective is a poignant example of an innovative strategy that has been implemented successfully to stimulate social change in an oppressed group. I conclude the chapter with some reflections on the lessons for emancipatory nursing that may be gained from the examination of this selection of foundational thought. Although I do not attempt to provide an exhaustive review of the philosophical underpinnings of emancipatory nursing here, it is my hope that this chapter will stimulate further reading and lively debate.

EMANCIPATORY NURSING

Nursing has been centrally concerned with health since Florence Nightingale (1859) declared that "true nursing" has to do with health, not disease. The move toward emancipatory nursing reflects changing views of health. For much of the twentieth century, health has been constructed as "the absence of disease or infirmity"—a biomedical view in which what causes disease is a determinant of health (Rachlis & Kushner, 1995; Registered Nurses' Association of British Columbia, 1992). In the 1970s, thinking on health broadened to include a behavioral approach. From this perspective, health incorporates the notion of physical well-being. Health determinants came to include lifestyle factors (Lalonde, 1974). Then, in the 1980s, with the introduction of the World Health Organization's Ottawa Charter for Health Promotion and related documents, socioenvironmental and population health approaches entered the popular domain (Green & Kreuter, 1991). According to these views, determinants of health include income, social status, education, food, a stable ecosystem, sustainable resources, and social justice and equity (World Health Organization, 1986). A composite view of health derived from these three perspectives is one of health as a multidimensional phenomenon involving interdependent physical, psychological, and sociopolitical dimensions (Capra, 1982; Evans & Stoddart, 1990). What does this mean for nursing?

Consistent with biomedical and behavioral views of health, models of nursing generally focus on physical and psychological dimensions of health, with little or no acknowledgment of broad sociopolitical dimensions such as poverty (Butterfield, 1990; Kendall, 1992). In turn, nursing research practices are traditionally based on empiricist models of research that are congruent with biomedical and behavioral views of health (Thompson, 1985; Webster & Jacox, 1985). Emancipatory nursing, with its emphasis on social inequalities, holds promise for solving problems relevant to population and socioenvironmental views of health. However, nurses working from this perspective clearly need to be involved politically. Furthermore, because the problems nurses confront in this realm of practice are highly value-laden (Webster

& Jacox, 1985), nurses need to develop ways of generating knowledge that are not traditionally viewed as value-free. Because emancipatory nursing calls nurses to take political action and requires that they use nontraditional research practices, continuity in the discipline is disrupted.

For nurses to move in this direction, understanding the philosophical roots behind the transformation from usual practices to new practices has the potential to demystify this transformation and thus empower nurses to act more cogently. The emancipatory project is placed within a broader context so that powerful factors acting on the change process can be identified and dealt with proactively.

Philosophical Foundations

Like any social phenomenon, emancipatory nursing is historically located relative to traditional social conventions and political ideologies (Benner, 1994; Kuhn, 1970; Laudan, 1977). Social practices such as nursing have more to do with what a society or community considers appropriate action than with a set of individual actions (Benner, 1994; Kuhn, 1970; Taylor, 1975). Professional practices are culturally constituted and thus have to do with shared meanings (Benner, 1994; Kuhn, 1970). Because common meanings are culturally dependent, and culture is constantly developing, the common meanings informing the science and practice of nursing are not static but ever changing and evolving. What foundational thought underlies the transformation from traditional nursing to emancipatory trends?

Roots of Modernity

Traditional approaches to nursing science and practice are the product of "modern" thought. Modern perspectives can be traced back to the seventeenth century, and since then they have dominated Western philosophical thought and scientific practices. However, there is a feeling that the modern period is coming to an end, with a move toward postmodern approaches to science (Bell, 1973). Understanding the character and boundaries of modern thought and locating emancipatory trends in nursing relative to this can be enlightening.

Nursing's roots can be traced back to Bacon, Descartes, and Locke, the founders of modernity (Borgmann, 1992; Capra, 1982). Bacon advocated systematic inquiry into phenomena to advance humankind's ability to dominate nature. Descartes explicated a systematic method to this end, and Locke fused the domination of nature with the primacy of method and the sovereignty of the individual (Borgmann, 1992). In 1627, Bacon wrote *New Atlantis,* in which he unleashed his dissatisfaction with the unprincipled and disorganized state of scientific inquiry. What is profound about Bacon's work is his shift from the perception of the earth and nature as a nurturing entity to the perception that nature must be dominated (Borgmann, 1992; Capra, 1982). Using violent and often vicious language, Bacon set out the terms of his new empirical method and instilled in modern science the value of control over nature, an outstanding example of the influence of patriarchal attitudes on scientific thought.

Descartes explicated Bacon's empirical method and proposed a method in which discovery and verification were pivotal. Descartes introduced the notion that method in science is preeminent (Borgmann, 1992; Capra, 1982). He put forward the idea of presenting thoughts in logical order, then systematically doubting the truth-value of those thoughts in order to identify those aspects of intuition that are true and those that are untrue (Cahn, 1977; Capra, 1982). Building on the work of Bacon and Descartes, Locke wrote *Treatise,* a celebration of the individual, which introduced the idea that the autonomy of the single self was the new authority (Borgmann, 1992). Thus the individual as the predominant unit of interest was instilled in modern science. Empirical science, method, and the individual were at the core of modernity. Modernity is characterized by three key dimensions: realism and its offspring, objectivity; belief in a universal law for human conduct that holds regardless of particular circumstances; and individualism and its adherent, autonomy (Borgmann, 1992).

Nightingale, the founder of modern nursing science, followed the scientific thinking of her time with regard to method, but diverged from the value of control over nature in her theoretical writings. To argue for change in the military hospital in Scutari, Nightingale compiled statistical data on health conditions in the army and used these data to write reports that identified areas for reform (Schuyler,

1992). In her theoretical writings, Nightingale posited that the reparative process is enhanced by allowing forces of nature to predominate, a position in opposition to the prevailing scientific value of the time that nature is a force to be dominated.

> The reparative process which Nature has instituted and which we call disease has been hindered by some want of knowledge or attention, in one or all of these things [fresh air, light, warmth, quiet, cleanliness, diet], and pain, suffering, or interruption of the whole [reparative] process sets in. (Nightingale, 1859, p. 5)

Thus, in theorizing that nature is indeed an ally and not a force to be dominated, Nightingale positioned nursing far from Baconian thought.

Advent of Postmodernism

Toward the close of the twentieth century, commanding critiques of realism and objectivity, universalism, and individualism have undermined the theoretical confidence and credibility of modernism (Borgmann, 1992). Critiques of modernism have been instrumental in exposing the limitations of modern approaches for developing knowledge with potential for meeting the needs of a democratic society in the face of cultural and moral crises of the late twentieth century (Borgmann, 1992; Capra, 1982; Gleick, 1987; Rorty, 1993). Critical and feminist theorists have been at the forefront of generating knowledge for social change relevant for late-twentieth-century society (Flax, 1988; Kincheloe & McLaren, 1994). With roots in the post-World War I German intellectual community, critical theory analyzes forms of domination (Kincheloe & McLaren, 1994). Arising from eighteenth-century scholarship, feminist theory focuses on the relationship between gender and patriarchal domination (Flax, 1988). The contributions of critical social theorists and feminists to emancipatory nursing are discussed in detail in other chapters within this volume.

Nursing theory influenced by modern perspectives is deemed inadequate in its capacity to reflect the reality with which it is supposedly concerned (Webster & Jacox, 1985). Postmodern perspectives offer an alternative approach to theory development for nursing. In particular, critical and feminist approaches to theory development are apparent in emancipatory nursing (Butterfield, 1990; Campbell & Bunting, 1991; Kendall, 1992). As previously mentioned, the goals of emancipatory nursing are "to help oppressed and disenfranchised persons gain freedom from the people, ideology, or situations that keep them oppressed" (Kendall, 1992, p. 2). However, emancipatory nursing operates within a social order (that is, a political ideology) that maintains the status quo for the benefit of dominant groups (Kendall, 1992). Explicating dimensions of the current social order has the potential to clarify the emancipatory project in nursing by revealing the underlying assumptions of the social order within which it is operating. Examining the critical discourse of Rousseau is enlightening to that end. Following is a brief overview of his political theory.

ROUSSEAU: AN INFLUENTIAL FOUNDER OF WESTERN SOCIAL ORDER

Western social order derives from classic political theory, drawing on the brilliance of such philosophers as Jean-Jacques Rousseau. Rousseau's political thought influenced the architects of the French and American revolutions, Marx and his followers, as well as thinkers as diverse and seminal as Tolstoy and Kant (Baradat, 1994; Luke, 1990; Rousseau, 1971). Thus Rousseau's work lives on in the minds of twentieth-century women and men. Born in Geneva, Rousseau was a highly influential eighteenth-century political philosopher who lived most of his life in France. His interpretation of such terms as *general will, freedom, government, law, sovereign,* and *citizen* continue to dominate modern political discourse (Baradat, 1994; Luke, 1990; Rousseau, 1978). Therefore, Rousseau's writings are foundational to the ideologies within which the emancipatory nursing project is embedded.

Much concerned with social order, Rousseau passionately and eloquently wrote several treatises in which his vision of and strategies for achieving a just society were characterized (Gay, 1983; Rousseau, 1978). In two highly influential political documents, *Discourse on the*

Origin and the Foundation of Inequality Among Mankind (1754) and *The Social Contract* (1762), Rousseau presented his view on the nature of man and his solution for establishing social order while ensuring freedom and "happiness" (see Rousseau, 1971).[1]

The Social Contract, a brilliant, original, and beautifully written book, articulates a distinct political philosophy (see Rousseau, 1954, 1978). An often-quoted paragraph introduces Rousseau's argument:

> Man was born free, but is everywhere in bondage. This or that man believes himself the master of his fellow men, but is nevertheless more of a slave than they. How did this change from freedom into bondage come about? I do not know. Under what conditions can it be rendered legitimate? This problem I believe I can solve. (Rousseau, 1983, p. 17)

Here Rousseau orients the reader to his central concerns: freedom and a just society. Rousseau believed that he had the answer, an answer outlined in *The Social Contract.*

According to Rousseau, harmony and cooperation can be achieved only through individual man's entering into a social contract with the state. Rousseau (1983) outlined the contractual basis of social obligation: "Each of us puts his person and all his power in common under the supreme direction of the general will; and in a body we receive each member as an indivisible part of the whole" (p. 24). According to Rousseau, a legitimate, just, political society can be attained through the abolishment of individual will. Individual will is sacrificed for the general will, the individual giving responsibility for social order over to the state: "This act of association produces a moral and collective body composed of as many members as there are voices in the assembly, which receives from its same act its unity, its common self, its life, and its will" (p. 24). What has puzzled philosophers about this formulation is the idea that giving over individual will to the general will is in some respects more liberating, not less so.

One influential philosopher who was intrigued by Rousseau's work was Immanuel Kant. Kant developed the relationship between freedom and will in his book *Groundwork of the Metaphysics of Morals* (1785/1956), in which he explicated the moral dimension of will: "A free will and will under moral laws are one and the same" (p. 114).

Much concerned with the relationship between duty and the good or moral will, Kant advanced the notion of a categorical imperative, an imperative that demands that one act morally, unconditionally. His most influential formulation ties the idea of moral action to general will: "Act only on that maxim whereby thou canst at the same time will that it should become universal law" (p. 88), meaning that, within a given context, any rational being would adopt that supreme principle. Kant held to the notion of a supreme principle, but concluded that the idea of a rational being is problematic. Interests, he pointed out, inevitably form the basis of the assumptions underlying human reason.

Rousseau also understood that "general will," as an abstraction, is problematic in practice because of private interests. He recognized that general will was often subverted by such interests:

> In the perfect legislation, the private or individual will should be null; the corporate will of the government very subordinate; and consequently the general or sovereign will always dominant and the unique rule of the others. According to the natural order, on the contrary, these different wills become more active as they are more concentrated. Thus, the general will is always the weakest, the corporate will has second place, and the private will is first of all. (Rousseau, 1983, p. 52)

Here, Rousseau points out that general will is in competition with corporate and private will. Further, he acknowledges the gap between theory and practice by identifying that the natural tendency of human nature is the reverse of the political principles he proposes. However, Rousseau missed a key point—women and minorities were not included as citizens (see Rousseau, 1971). Rousseau's "general will" therefore represented only the collective will of men of the assembly. For Rousseau, the assembly was the governing body of the community, the sole function of which was to carry out the wishes of the community (general will) (Baradat, 1994).

Examination of Rousseau's political theory, as delineated in *The Social Contract* and further explored by Kant, is foundational for inquiry concerning social action because it compels us to rethink the fundamental ideas that are conventionally used to justify action or inaction and to examine the context within which these ideas are articulated (Rousseau, 1978). Particularly relevant for emancipatory nursing is the notion of "will" and the related notion of "interests." Rousseau proposed a widely adopted theory for social order that was based on the notion of equitable relationships. But in practice, interests intrude, creating tensions among general, corporate, and private will, leading to a climate governed by hidden agendas in which dominant interests prevail (Rousseau, 1971). Unmasking hidden, age-old social conventions that maintain inequitable relationships is central to the emancipatory project. Outstanding examples of disclosing moral and social conventions that contribute to relationships of oppression can be found in the work of Marx, Freire, and Habermas.

MARX, FREIRE, AND HABERMAS: CONSTRUCTING THEORIES FOR SOCIAL CHANGE

Karl Marx was a philosopher of modern times whose thoughts have had worldwide impact on knowledge development and social change (Baradat, 1994; Marx & Engels, 1959). Further, scholars in all fields of human knowledge have been influenced by Marx's writings (see Marx, 1964; Marx & Engels, 1959). Like Rousseau, Marx was concerned with the rights of man and the notion of freedom. What remains as an enduring contribution is Marx's argument for the primacy of economics in shaping history. Economic determinism, in which the primary human motivation is economic, is a fundamental assumption of Marx's sociological theory (Baradat, 1994). Marx viewed societies as consisting of two parts: the foundational and the superstructure. The foundational consists of resources and technologies that are society's means of production as well as the relations of production, that is, owners and workers. The superstructure consists of all nonmaterial institutions in society, such as art, law, religion, ideology, education, government, and values. According to this theory, the function of the superstructure is to assure that the owners remain in positions of dominance and that workers are kept in their place (Baradat, 1994). This is accomplished through the inculcation in people of society's dominant values and norms to the benefit of dominant groups. Here, Marx demonstrated how Rousseau's strategy for equality had gone awry: Individual will is shaped by society for the benefit of dominant groups. Thus Marx identified and named the dynamics of economically dependent power relationships.

Marx carried his argument of economically dependent power relationships over to the arena of science, one of the domains of the superstructure. He revealed the social character of science, arguing that the shape and success of modern science can be linked to the interests of capital in its quest to develop modern commerce and industry (Bernal, 1952). Marx's views on science have been further developed for the emancipatory project by critical social theorists.

Marx's crowning contribution was his linking of thought with action. In the *Theses on Feuerbach XI* (1846), he states, "Philosophers have only interpreted their world in various ways: The point is to change it" (Marx, 1975, p. 423). He labeled the testing of theories in the real world *praxis.* Marx's theories, put into practice, have made possible what was impossible for 20 centuries—a level of freedom from exploitation through programs such as social security, pensions, paid holidays, unions, and scholarships (Baradat, 1994; Marx & Engels, 1959). Marx thereby established that linking thought with action is a powerful catalyst for social change. Conceptual direction for emancipatory nursing can be found in the work of Marx, particularly in relation to conceptualizing economically dependent power relationships and in relation to developing the notion of praxis for nursing.

Marxian praxis was further developed by Paulo Freire in the 1960s. Freire, who experienced the debilitating effects of poverty as a youth in Latin America, committed his life to a struggle against forces maintaining conditions of poverty. In 1970, he wrote *Pedagogy of the Oppressed,* in which he drew on the work of a wide range of scholars and philosophers to uncover what he called the "culture of silence" of the dispossessed. Thus he shifted responsibility for the ignorance and lethargy evident in the deprived to the economic, social, and political domination of which they were the victims. Freire advanced the notions that every human being is capable of looking critically at the world in which she or he is immersed and that this critical appraisal is facilitated by dialogical encounter with others.

In so doing, Freire upset a fundamental aspect of the social order—individuals living in deprived circumstances were encouraged to voice their will, not alone, but with each other. Thus the deprived had the opportunity to uncover a collective will that existed in opposition to the dominant view. Then, aspects of the hidden agenda that supported those in positions of power could be identified and articulated. Once aspects of the hidden agenda became evident, the focus for action was clear and steps to make change could be identified and implemented. Not only did Freire propose a theory for social change, but integral to the theory was an action component directed at the very heart of the philosophy bolstering the existing social order. Of his work, he writes: "This work deals with a very obvious truth: just as the oppressor, in order to oppress needs a theory of oppressive action, so the oppressed in order to become free, also need a theory of action . . . only in the encounter of the people with their revolutionary leaders—in their . . . praxis—can this theory be built" (p. 185). From Freire's work, emancipatory nursing can conceptualize both a strategy for working with the oppressed, the dialogical encounter, and a role, working with the oppressed to build theory.

Jürgen Habermas, a critical theorist who wrote in the 1960s, extended Marx's work by casting old problems in a new light (Held, 1980). Habermas was centrally concerned with knowledge production for social change. For Habermas (1971), knowledge is historically rooted and interest bound: "The only knowledge that can truly orient action is knowledge that frees itself from mere human interests and is based on Ideas—in other words, knowledge that has taken a theoretical attitude" (p. 301). Building his version of a critical theory, Habermas drew on disparate traditions of scholarship, including Marxian theory, symbolic interactionism (Mead), role theory (Parsons), and cognitive developmental psychology (Kohlberg, Piaget) (Habermas, 1970; Held, 1980). For Habermas, as for other critical theorists and feminists, it is action that counts.

A central issue identified by Habermas is that technocratic consciousness justifies a particular class interest in domination and affects the very structure of human interests (Habermas, 1973; Held, 1980). Habermas (1971) offered a theory for making visible what he calls "knowledge-constitutive interests": technical-cognitive interests, which relate to interest in control; practical interests, which relate to meaning construction within a normative order; and emancipatory or critical interests, identifying theoretical statements that express ideologically frozen relations of dependence that can in principle be transformed.

Habermas proposed a critical methodology. Here, the dual strategies of reflection and dialogue are directed toward examining the three interests featured in Habermas's theory: technical, practical, and emancipatory (Habermas, 1971). Reflection on and discussion about technical interests involve examining who has authority and how technical interests shape reality (Allen, 1987). Reflection on and discussion of practical interests involve determining by what standards the facts are constituted (Habermas, 1971). Emancipatory interest involves reflecting on and discussing whether or not theoretical statements are an accurate reflection of social action or represent ideologically frozen relationships. The goal of such reflection and discussion, Habermas (1971) explained, is to unite knowledge and interest in a "dialectic that takes the historical traces of suppressed dialogue and reconstructs what has been suppressed" (p. 315). Habermas suggested an approach that can be used by emancipatory nursing to identify whose interests are served in situations of oppression.

SIGNIFICANCE OF SOCIAL CHANGE THEORIES FOR EMANCIPATORY NURSING

What is gained by reflecting on the foundational knowledge for the emancipatory project of nursing? Knowledge development in nursing is traditionally constructed from the perspective of modern thought, which is embedded in a social order that perpetuates dominant interests. Focus on the individual, a tendency toward realism and universalism, has produced knowledge that serves the dominant interests by expressing ideologically frozen relationships of dependence and by silencing the oppressed. In the past two decades, postmodern critiques have uncovered how the tenets of modern thought contribute to maintaining the status quo, thereby undermining the confidence and credibility of the modern project (Borgmann, 1992). However, few theorists have identified how to develop knowledge for transforming relationships of dependence (Borgmann, 1992). Marx, Freire, and Habermas are exceptions; they have proposed strategies and theories that can be further developed by nursing toward knowledge for social change. Marx advanced a theory for uncovering the dynamics of economically dependent relationships and introduced the notion of praxis, a strategy that links thought and action in an iterative process directed toward social change to benefit the oppressed. Freire proposed a theory for social change that was action oriented as well and introduced a strategy for working with the oppressed to create change, the dialogical encounter. Habermas was much concerned with ideologically frozen relations of dependence and envisioned an approach that linked reflection and discussion as means of examining and reconstructing what is suppressed. Emancipatory nursing practice and inquiry informed by foundational thought on social change have the potential to evolve in an informed and theoretically sound manner by drawing on a strong theoretical foundation.

CONCLUSION

With increasing awareness of the role that social inequities play in health, there is an emphasis on nursing practice directed toward reducing social inequities and a related move toward developing methods for research and inquiry that are useful for producing relevant knowledge. This is referred to as emancipatory nursing, a direction that involves social action to reduce inequalities for the benefit of oppressed groups. In working with the oppressed to reduce social inequalities, nursing, once comfortably aligned with dominant groups, is now in opposition to them—a significant shift in perspective. Great thinkers such as Rousseau, Marx, Freire, and, more recently, Habermas have long been concerned with social inequalities. Drawing on foundational knowledge for social change such as that produced by these theorists, emancipatory nursing can begin to make significant contributions toward health.

NOTE

1. Because Rousseau was referring only to persons of the male gender in his writing, use of the word *man* and male pronouns in reference to his work is appropriate.

REFERENCES

Allen, D. G. (1987). Critical social theory as a model for analyzing ethical issues in family and community health. *Family Community Health, 10,* 63-72.

Baradat, L. P. (1994). *Political ideologies: Their origins and impact* (5th ed.). Englewood Cliffs, NJ: Prentice Hall.

Bell, D. (1973). *The coming of post-industrial society: A venture in social forecasting.* New York: Basic Books.

Benner, P. (1994). The role of articulation in understanding practice and experience as sources of knowledge in clinical nursing. In J. Tully (Ed.), *Philosophy in an age of pluralism* (pp. 136-158). Cambridge, UK: Cambridge University Press.

Bernal, J. D. (1952). *Marx and science.* New York: International.

Borgmann, A. (1992). *Crossing the postmodern divide.* Chicago: University of Chicago Press.

Butterfield, P. (1990). Thinking upstream: Nurturing a conceptual understanding of the societal context of health behavior. *Advances in Nursing Science, 12*(2), 1-8.

Cahn, S. (Ed.). (1977). *Classics of Western philosophy.* Indianapolis, IN: Hackett.

Campbell, J. C., & Bunting, S. (1991). Voices and paradigms: Perspectives on critical and feminist theory in nursing. *Advances in Nursing Science, 13*(3), 1-15.

Capra, F. (1982). *The turning point: Science, society and the rising culture.* New York: Simon & Schuster.

Evans, R., & Stoddart, G. L. (1990). Producing health consuming health care. *Social Science and Medicine, 31,* 1347-1364.

Flax, J. (1988). Beyond equality: Gender, justice and difference. In G. Bock & S. James (Eds.), *Beyond equality and difference: Citizenship, feminist politics, female subjectivity* (pp. 193-210). New York: Routledge.

Freire, P. (1970). *Pedagogy of the oppressed.* New York: Continuum.

Gay, P. (1983). Introduction. In J.-J. Rousseau, *On the social contract; Discourse on the origin of inequality; Discourse on political economy* (D. A. Cress, Ed. & Trans.) (pp. 1-12). Indianapolis, IN: Hackett.

Gleick, J. (1987). *Chaos theory: Making a new science.* New York: Penguin.

Green, L. W., & Kreuter, M. (1991). *Health promotion planning: An educational and environmental approach.* Toronto: Mayfield.

Habermas, J. (1970). *Towards a rational society: Student protest, science, and politics* (J. J. Shapiro, Trans.). London: Heinemann.

Habermas, J. (1971). *Knowledge and human interests* (J. J. Shapiro, Trans.). London: Heinemann.

Habermas, J. (1973). *Theory and practice* (J. Viertel, Trans.). Boston: Beacon.

Held, D. (1980). *Introduction to critical social theory.* London: Hutchinson.

Kant, I. (1956). *Groundwork of the metaphysics of morals* (H. J. Paton, Ed.). New York: Harper & Row. (Original work published 1785)

Kendall, J. (1992). Fighting back: Promoting emancipatory nursing actions. *Advances in Nursing Science, 15*(2), 1-15.

Kincheloe, J. L., & McLaren, P. L. (1994). Rethinking critical theory and qualitative research. In N. K. Denzin & Y. S. Lincoln (Eds.), *Handbook of qualitative research* (pp. 138-157). Thousand Oaks, CA: Sage.

Kuhn, T. (1970). *The structure of scientific revolutions* (2nd ed.). Chicago: University of Chicago Press.

Lalonde, M. (1974). *New perspectives on the health of Canadians.* Ottawa: Health and Welfare Canada.

Laudan, L. (1977). *Progress and its problems: Toward a theory of scientific growth.* Berkeley: University of California Press.

Luke, T. W. (1990). *Social theory and modernity: Critique, dissent, and revolution.* Newbury Park, CA: Sage.

Marx, K. (1964). *Early writings* (T. B. Bottomore, Ed.). New York: McGraw-Hill.

Marx, K. (1975). *Early writings* (Q. Hoare, Ed.). New York: Vintage.

Marx, K., & Engels, F. (1959). *Basic writings on politics and philosophy* (L. Feuer, Ed.). Garden City, NY: Anchor.

Ministry of Supply and Services Canada. (1994). *Strategies for population health: Investing in the health of Canadians.* Ottawa: Health Canada.

Moccia, P. (1988). At the fault line: Social activism and caring. *Nursing Outlook, 36*, 30-33.

Nightingale, F. (1859). *Notes on nursing: What it is, and what it is not.* London: Harrison.

Rachlis, M., & Kushner, C. (1995). *Strong medicine.* Toronto: HarperCollins.

Registered Nurses' Association of British Columbia. (1992). *Determinants of health: Empowering strategies for nursing practice.* Vancouver: Author.

Rorty, R. (1993). *Philosophical papers: Vol. 1. Objectivity, relativism, and truth.* New York: Cambridge University Press.

Rousseau, J.-J. (1954). *The social contract* (W. Kendall, Ed.). Chicago: Gateway.

Rousseau, J.-J. (1971). *The social contract and discourse on the origin of inequality* (L. G. Crocker, Ed.). New York: Washington Square.

Rousseau, J.-J. (1978). *On the social contract* (R. D. Masters, Ed., & J. R. Masters, Trans.). New York: St. Martin's.

Rousseau, J.-J. (1983). *On the social contract; Discourse on the origin of inequality; Discourse on political economy* (D. A. Cress, Ed. & Trans.). Indianapolis, IN: Hackett.

Schuyler, C. (1992). Florence Nightingale. In F. Nightingale, *Notes on nursing: What it is and what it is not* (D. P. Carrol, Ed.) (Commemorative ed., pp. 3-17). Philadelphia: J. B. Lippincott.

Taylor, C. (1975). *Hegel.* Cambridge, UK: Cambridge University Press.

Thompson, J. (1985). Practical discourse in nursing: Going beyond empiricism and historicism. *Advances in Nursing Science, 7*(4), 59-71.

Webster, G., & Jacox, A. (1985). The liberation of nursing theory. In J. C. McCloskey & H. K. Grace (Eds.), *Current issues in nursing* (2nd ed., pp. 21-29). Boston: Blackwell Scientific.

World Health Organization. (1986). Ottawa Charter for Health Promotion. *Health Promotion, 1*(4), 3-5.

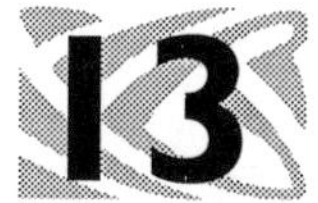

Nursing Inquiry for the Common Good

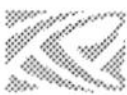

ROSALIE STARZOMSKI
PATRICIA RODNEY

Nurse theorists are engaged increasingly in reflection on the philosophical foundations of nursing. Much of this reflection has paralleled changes in the philosophy of science as revolutions (or evolutions) in the paradigms of science have become visible in diverse fields of human inquiry (Kuhn, 1970; Laudan, 1977). Through their inquiry, nurses stand on the threshold of making important contributions to knowledge for practice, or praxis (Allen, 1992; Bunting & Campbell, 1994). This means that nursing knowledge "can be used as a sociopolitical power to enforce a theorized good and to effect human health in unforeseeable ways" (Reed, 1989, p. 8).

However, nurses are not over the threshold. As we examine the development of nursing theory and nursing ethics, we find that the focus has been on individual patients and their family members, and the responsibilities of nurses toward these persons, with little attention to the social, political, and economic contexts of health and health care. Until recently, there has been limited direction from nursing theory to attend to that context. If we assume that theories direct practice and that there are essential links among theory, practice, and research, this means that nursing research and practice have traditionally neglected the social, political, and economic contexts of health and health care. This is problematic in an applied discipline such as nursing, where the ultimate test of theories is the usefulness of the ideas in the real world, where patients and practitioners interact (Donaldson, 1995; Thorne, 1993).

In this chapter, we make the case for expansion of social, environmental, and political thinking in nursing inquiry. This means that we call for those of us in nursing to extend our focus to encompass the well-being of the aggregate, or the common good, in our theoretical and empirical work. We will argue that an important goal of our profession should be to ensure that our inquiry has an impact on the development of health policy for the common good—a goal that requires attention to interdisciplinary work as well as work within our own profession. In developing our argument, we begin with a discussion of professional responsibilities, which we follow with a commentary about directions for nursing theory and nursing ethics.

PROFESSIONAL RESPONSIBILITIES AS CONTEXT

Unique obligations befall all health care professionals, including nurses, because their prudence is called upon to help steer patients' lives. This means that health care professionals must exercise their specialized judgment and skill for the good of patients (Sokolowski, 1991). Given the trust that patients must put in professionals, professional-patient relationships may be characterized as fiduciary—that is, based on trust or fidelity (May, 1989).

Upholding trust and fidelity in an era of health care reform and cost constraint is, however, problematic. To illustrate, in a qualitative study completed by the first author, in which emergency nurses' perceptions of the ethical issues encountered in their practice were described, nurses identified multiple and complex problems related to access to health care. Portrayals of patients lined up waiting in the halls of emergency departments with minimal care available, or being discharged with inadequate home care or other support, were common. As one nurse related:

> A lot of people come in, quote, "as placement problems," and it used to be that a placement problem simply meant that somebody was elderly and what they needed was a nursing home, and there was always a shortage of that. . . . Now the kinds of placement problems we're seeing [are] patients being discharged into the community with much more complex situations, and I don't believe that there's the . . . access to . . . [the necessary] facilities out in the community. . . . We're seeing patients coming in that are much more acutely ill than they ever used to be, but they're being discharged still relatively acutely ill.

Nurses' descriptions of the lack and/or fragmentation of services for clients with mental health problems were particularly alarming. As another nurse said:

> Probably one of the most frustrating things to me is knowing that someone is in need of mental health follow-up. . . . They're being sent home from Emergency. It's not satisfactory to me to have them return to the same situations that caused them to be depressed and suicidal in the beginning. . . . There's so many holes that people fall through the cracks.

In our experience, the concerns voiced by these nurses are not isolated. We have encountered instances in which health care cutbacks have had direct impacts on patient care. For example, the first author was involved in a lobbying campaign (eventually successful) against a decision that was made by one Canadian province to cut universal funding for immunosuppression medication taken by transplant recipients to prevent organ rejection. With many people in need of such medication unable to pay for it, the funding cut could lead to some persons' not taking their drugs, experiencing rejection of their transplanted organs, and, in some cases, dying as a result of the government's shortsighted decision.

Thus research and experience support current warnings that problems of access to health care are growing at an alarming pace (Rachlis & Kushner, 1994; Watson, 1994). At the same time, we are aware that the broader determinants of health (e.g., economic and employment cycles and educational opportunities) are poorly understood (Evans, 1994). Problems of access to health care violate the ethical principles of fidelity and justice (Morreim, 1988). Although we know that there is a need for the development of equitable services for diverse groups of people whose voices may not have been heard previously in the development of health policy (Anderson, Blue, & Lau, 1991; Sherwin, 1992; Thorne, 1993), there is evidence that some of these groups are even more at risk from current cost constraint measures (Bunting, 1992; Ericksen, Rodney, & Starzomski, 1995; Kjellstrand, 1992; Watson, 1994). For instance, in a recent study by a Canadian provincial nurses' association, nurses reported serious situations of neglect of the elderly in nursing homes, early discharge of patients, failure to admit patients to hospitals because of lack of beds or inadequate assessment, and inadequate staffing in acute psychiatric areas (Oberle & Grant, 1994).

All of this underscores the urgent need for nursing theory, research, and practice to address the social, political, and economic contexts of health and health care. In order to address these contexts, we need to think about our professional responsibilities at three different levels: the micro level, or the level of individual professional responsibilities for patients and families under our care; the meso level, or the level of institutional responsibilities for programs of care; and the macro level, or the level of societal responsibilities for the health of the total population (Rodney & Starzomski, 1994; Yeo, 1993). Most health care professionals, including nurses, have tended to focus on the micro and, to a lesser extent, meso levels. Given the problems of access to health care faced by our patients and their family members, one of our most immediate challenges is to expand our work at the macro level. This requires that we understand and promote the common good.

THE COMMON GOOD

Trust and fidelity have been articulated primarily at the micro level of professional responsibilities to individual patients and their family members. Consequently, health care professionals have tended traditionally to ignore their public duties (Danis & Churchill, 1991; Jennings, Callahan, & Wolf, 1987). Within nursing, we are beginning to realize that to integrate equitable access to health care as a valued research and practice goal, we need to move beyond conceptualizing at the individual level and instead theoretically frame access in its broadest sociopolitical context (Bridges & Lynam, 1993; Jones & Meleis, 1993; Stevens, 1992). Portnoy and Dumas (1994), for instance, remind us that "nursing for the public good in the 1990's . . . involves negotiating a more fragmented and complex health care system and a more complex and populous world" (p. 374).

What Portnoy and Dumas describe as nursing for the public good can be understood in terms of the *public interest* and the *common good.* As Jennings et al. (1987) explain:

> Service that promotes the public interest includes the professions' contribution of technical expertise to public policy analysis, and indirect service to society that is a byproduct of service to individual members of society. Service that promotes the common good includes the distinctive and critical perspective the various professions have to offer on basic human values, and on facets of the human good and the good life. It also includes the professions' contribution to what may be called civic discourse or public philosophy—that ongoing, pluralistic conversation in a democratic society about our shared goals, our common purposes, and the nature of the good life in a just social order. (p. 6)

We believe that our professional responsibilities at the micro and meso levels of the health care system primarily serve the public interest, whereas our responsibilities at the macro level focus on promoting the common good. Given the concerns we discussed earlier about the impact of health care cuts, nurses must become more proactive in pluralistic conversations about shared goals and common purposes in terms of access to health services and the broader determinants of health. This requires that we add to the formulation of substantive goals by contributing to empirical and theoretical work on social justice (Aroskar, 1992). It also requires that we participate in a process of social advocacy so that we may respond to the needs of underserved people and society at large (Fowler, 1990). To do this, we must reflect on nursing theory and on the relationship of nursing theory to nursing ethics. This will provide theoretical direction for our research so that we may prepare ourselves to participate in the formulation of just public policy.

NURSING THEORY AND NURSING ETHICS

Nursing Inquiry

Both scientific and philosophical inquiry in nursing are required if we are to reflect on nursing theory and on the relationship of nursing theory to nursing ethics. Scientific inquiry helps us to understand the "is" of the empirical world, whereas philosophical inquiry helps us to understand the "ought" (Jameton & Fowler, 1989). More specifically, philosophical inquiry includes a focus on epistemology (what we know and how we know it), feminist and other critiques of the philosophy of science, and professional ethics (Fry, 1992). Although our primary purpose in this chapter is to focus on the last of these, we wish to commence by locating what we have to say in terms of epistemology and the philosophy of science.

Many of the revolutions/evolutions in the paradigms of science that nursing finds itself a part of have been based on an epistemology that rejects the traditional belief in objective, rational foundations to all knowledge (Luke & Gore, 1992). This epistemology has been defined as naturalized and results in questions of fact (descriptive inquiry) being relevant to questions about value (normative inquiry) (Kornblith, 1985). What this means is that the epistemological assumptions behind some of the newer paradigms of science allow for a reciprocity of facts and values. Science is no longer considered to be "objective," but is understood to be value-laden. We have come to understand that we should see scientific progress as a historical process, and should hold up for question the (usually implicit) values that have driven it. Moreover, we can look to the facts provided by science to move us toward decisions about normative goals. Within the philosophy of science, we thus find ourselves in a postmodern state.

It is important to note that the changes brought about by a postmodern epistemology are not unproblematic. Squires (1993) warns that "although liberating, and even democratizing, in its refusal of hierarchy and certainty, the postmodern condition is paralyzing in its deconstruction of all 'principled positions' " (p. 1). What does this mean for nursing inquiry? As we see it, the focus of nursing inquiry should no longer be merely on the control of phenomena of concern *or* the interpretation of the meaning of human experience; nursing inquiry should focus on the generation of emancipatory social change (Allen, 1992; Anderson, 1991; Campbell & Bunting, 1991). As Reed (1995) explains:

> Nursing knowledge development need not abandon completely modernist views about high theory or universal ideals. Rather than capitulate entirely to postmodernism, nurses can knowingly involve in their science the realm of perspectives and values . . . that distinguish nursing knowledge and the caring application of that knowledge. (p. 76)

Critical theoretical perspectives (for example, critical social theory and feminist theory) are increasingly evident in nursing inquiry. We believe that such critical perspectives are able to take us from the "is" to the "ought" and thereby provide normative direction for change. We see this as a "weak form of postmodernism" (Squires, 1993, p. 12), where we can attend to the meaning of human experience while still arguing for the promotion of normative goals such as social justice and the common good.

The Relationship of Nursing Theory to Nursing Ethics

Although there is controversy about what constitutes nursing theory, it is not our purpose to enter into the debate here. We are assuming that there are levels of theory, and that each of these levels is required for practice. Furthermore, we are assuming that theories direct practice, and that there are links among theory, research, and practice such that the three may be considered as a triad, intricately connected and dependent on one another (Hathaway & Strong, 1988; Meleis, 1991). Theories direct practice by providing statements that may predict and control the phenomena with which nurses are concerned, serving as a basis for decision making. In contrast, nursing practice often yields insights into phenomena and uncovers gaps in existing theories (Hathaway & Strong, 1988). The research component of the triad validates theories' abilities to describe, explain, predict, and control. This becomes a reciprocal, interrelated, and continuously evolving process.

Whereas there is controversy about what constitutes nursing theory, there has been only preliminary thought about what constitutes nursing ethics (Fry, 1989; Penticuff, 1991). This preliminary thought has included questions about the place of ethical principles in nursing, the role of an ethic of care, the nature of patient-professional relationships, and characteristics of nurses as moral agents (Cooper, 1988; Fry, 1989, 1992; Liaschenko, 1993). Despite a lack of consensus on what nursing theory and nursing ethics *are*, a number of theorists agree that the development of nursing theory and nursing ethics needs to be more explicitly linked (Fry, 1992; Reed, 1989; Yeo, 1989). We concur with this position. As Reed (1989) explains, "Ethical inquiry into one's conceptual frame can provide needed constraints on the human tendency to blur the distinction between a researcher's beliefs and societal needs and can also provide the moral vision needed to effectively and humanely solve nursing problems" (p. 8).

How to link the development of nursing theory and nursing ethics is a more difficult issue than *whether* the two should be linked. Given our focus within this chapter on professional responsibilities at the macro level (with our corresponding call for promotion of the common good), we would like to suggest that we should start by broadening our theoretical mandate and adopting a normative stance. Broadening our theoretical mandate requires a reexamination of nursing's domain of knowledge,[1] and the adoption of a normative stance requires an explicit commitment to emancipatory health policy.

MOVING BEYOND RHETORIC TOWARD THE COMMON GOOD

Reexamining Nursing's Domain

Within nursing's domain of knowledge, we will address the major concepts of the client and the environment. Our focus will be on the environment, but we wish to start by noting two concerns about the client of nursing. First, the concept of the client requires expansion to provide direction to consider the needs of the aggregate as well as the individual (Fry, 1985; Storch, 1986). In other words, the client of nursing needs to be inclusive of individuals, families, citizens, and communities as active participants in health care planning at the individual and societal levels. Second, we are aware that the notion of "client" has been criticized by feminist and other theorists for carrying an individualistic bias and for overlooking systemic inequities—all "clients" do not have equal opportunities to be active participants (Sherwin, 1992). In order to address both of these concerns, nursing needs to focus on the environment within which the client is located.

Although environment has been said to be an important concept in the domain of nursing, its definition remains ambiguous, resulting in a growing recognition that the concept needs to be reexamined and expanded (Kleffel, 1991a, 1991b). Nurse theorists have viewed the concept of environment in a number of different ways, depending on the paradigmatic origins of their models (Meleis, 1991). The environment has been viewed primarily either as the immediate surroundings or circumstances of the individual or family or as an interactional field to which individuals adapt, adjust, or conform (Chopoorian, 1986). Because of this focus, most of the nursing research examining the environment has focused on the patient, the family, or the nurse (Kleffel, 1991b).

There has been a recent move to reexamine the concept of environment, with a number of authors suggesting expansion from the immediate milieu to which clients must respond and adapt to the broader societal context (Kleffel, 1991b; Stevens, 1989). Chopoorian

(1986) has expressed surprise that nurses are not more involved in the problems that result from situations within the environment. She posits that the lack of consciousness related to environment may contribute to the peripheral role of nursing in social, economic, and political affairs, and she challenges nurses to broaden their conception of the environment from the client-oriented psychosocial paradigm to sociopolitical economic concepts. Kleffel (1991a) proposes the need for an ecofeminist perspective on the environment. She suggests that nursing (as a primarily female profession) and the environment share a long history of domination and oppression and that an ecofeminist perspective would offer a conceptual foundation for developing a new consciousness of the environment with the potential for liberating both. Furthermore, Butterfield (1990) proposes an "upstream" nursing approach that focuses on modifying economic, political, and environmental factors that are seen as precursors of poor health, as opposed to the more conventional "downstream" approach, in which the individual is the locus of change.

Nurses involved in examining critical social theory also call for expansion of the concept of environment. Stevens (1989) discusses a framework in which nurses can reconceptualize their understanding of environment to encompass social, political, and economic constraints upon health. She suggests that "critical social reconceptualization of the environment involves uncovering and critiquing the oppressive social structures that constrain persons' health, limit their life possibilities, and restrict their equal and fully conscious participation in society" (p. 63). She goes on to assert that the more accurately and extensively individuals are able to perceive and reflect upon their social, political, and economic environment, the more effective they become in interaction with the environment, a condition that is the essence of health (p. 63).

In summary, several nurse theorists provide significant direction for the development of major concepts that can be used to develop and change the system in which care is delivered. Their direction helps us to broaden our theoretical mandate through a reexamination of nursing's domain of knowledge. This is necessary but not sufficient to promote the common good. We also require an explicit commitment to emancipatory health policy.

Emancipatory Health Policy

In the current health care system, nurses are involved not only in providing care to individuals and their families, but in advocating for, and assisting with, the development of health policy that affects groups of health care consumers. However, the idea of including health policy as a topic is a relatively new concept in modern nursing curricula. Nursing literature on the topic was almost nonexistent even 20 years ago (Fagin, 1981). At that time, there was little interest in research or theory building related to health care delivery in any of the disciplines and in the nursing literature in particular (Kos-Munson, 1992). Neither nurse theorists nor nursing curriculum developers identified health policy development as an area of focus (Lefort, 1993; Stevens, 1992). Milio (1984) suggests not only that nurses should be involved in influencing health policy, but that nurses need to move beyond this to influence policy making and to develop alternative policies that will effect an influence on the system. In light of the major challenges facing us in the areas of resource allocation and health care reform, several authors advocate nurses' greater involvement in these areas (Gillis, 1992; Stevens, 1992).

Not only is there a paucity of information in the nursing theory and education literature about health policy and the health care system, there is also little nursing research in the area. Although recently there have been recommendations about the need for health policy research in nursing, few studies have been conducted that have had significant impacts on public policy (Nagelkerk & Henry, 1991; Raudonis & Griffith, 1991). Nagelkerk and Henry (1991) suggest that good policy studies are needed that address the fundamental social problems on which nurses are most likely to have the greatest impact. Ingersoll, Hoffart, and Schultz (1990), who reviewed health services research in nursing, conclude that studies pertaining to health care technology, information systems, and ethical decision making are notably missing. They identify exploratory and descriptive studies of ethical issues related to use of scarce resources and the creation of ethical environments for care delivery as areas that require nursing research. Ingersoll et al. also suggest that the ethics of allocation of limited resources cannot be studied separately from issues of quality of care delivery, quality of patient outcomes, use of technology, human resources, cost-benefit analyses, and productivity in the health care arena, because these are so interrelated and interdependent.

Although there are gaps in the theory and research components of the theory-research-practice triad, there are many practice domain areas in which nurses have been involved actively in health care reform and health policy development. This involvement has been increasing over the past 15 years in both Canada and the United States (Curtin, 1993; Larsen & Baumgart, 1992; Lefort, 1993). Because of this, Curtin (1993) predicts that "nurses and nursing leaders will have greater impact on health policy development—and greater opportunity to develop new roles—than at any time since Florence Nightingale" (p. 8).

Social Activism

We have argued that we require an explicit commitment to emancipatory health policy in promoting the common good. Translating that commitment into action necessitates social activism—a route of social expression that Kendall (1992) claims has not been used by nurses on a major scale since the early days of modern nursing history. In fact, Moccia (1988) advocates a return to the approach to nursing as practiced by early nurse leaders and health care reformers such as Florence Nightingale, Lillian Wald, Margaret Sanger, and Lavinia Dock. Both Kendall and Moccia assert that nursing has been involved more recently with helping people adapt to their oppression than with helping them to gain freedom from it.

Moccia (1988) further notes that, because of the crisis we are facing in health care, nursing's tradition of caring and radical change are needed now more than ever before. One of the reasons cited for the slow growth of health promotion over the years has been the lack of attention to contextual influences on either health or behavior—areas that nurses such as Nightingale identified many years ago. Williams (1991) states that one way to express nurses' caring about health is to encourage and organize citizen groups to become involved in political advocacy for health, reinforcing once again that nurses have to extend their focus to look more broadly at the contexts in which people live in order to initiate emancipatory change.

Clearly, there are multiple arenas where explicit links between the development of nursing theory and nursing ethics can provide nurses with direction for social activism. For instance, nurses care for the victims of family violence and violent crime. Would not a focus on lobbying against the use of firearms and violence in our society be an appropriate direction for nursing to take? And what about nursing input into public policies that have a profound impact on how care is provided—for example, policies related to assisted suicide, informed consent, and advance directives? Decisions about issues such as building, closing, or expanding hospitals and moving to regional models of health delivery become ethical concerns as conflicting values and considerations are weighed. Nursing theory must direct us to consider the moral and ethical components of care delivery if it is to be useful for practicing nurses, and if our profession is to make a difference in promoting the common good.

Knowledge Production and Dissemination

As theory is developed, research is needed to examine its application in the practice setting. More nursing and interdisciplinary research is required in the health policy arena, with a view to improving patient care and health outcomes. As society is being called on to make choices in regard to resource allocation at the micro, meso, and macro levels, nursing is challenged to conduct research that focuses on ways to enhance moral reasoning, moral sensitivity, and moral accountability in the health policy arena. We require more knowledge about how these choices are being made (descriptive theory) to provide direction for how they should be made (normative theory). A qualitative study currently being conducted by this chapter's first author illustrates such an initiative. It draws on consumer and health care provider focus group data to examine stakeholder opinions about ethical issues in organ transplantation, with a view to uncovering how various members of society make decisions about difficult issues such as resource allocation. It is our hope that the results of such work will provides direction for health policy development.

In addition to developing nursing research and theory, it is imperative that we expand nursing program curricula to include more theoretical content about leadership, social and health care reform, and health policy in order to provide direction for these new demands upon nursing practice. It is essential for nursing faculty to shift their focus toward helping students to develop methods for influencing change within the health care system.

CONCLUSION

We have argued here for an expansion of social, environmental, and political thinking in nursing, calling upon a focus on the well-being of the aggregate, or the common good, in our theoretical and empirical work. We thus concur with Moccia's (1988) claim that intervention by nursing in sociopolitical structures is as essential to promoting health and preventing illness as are nurses' activities with individual clients.

Our inquiry must have an impact on the development of health policy for the common good—as we stated at the outset, a goal that requires attention to interdisciplinary work as well as work within our own profession. We therefore emphasize the need for more interdisciplinary approaches to education, research, and practice in order to break down barriers related to social reform so that we can work to improve the population's health status. Nurses are not the only professionals examining their models of practice and theory. Although it is important to develop theory for nursing practice, we should be cognizant that our theory may overlap with that of other disciplines, where goals for patient care are similar to our own and where calls for health care reform and resulting health policy are also inextricably linked with theory development and ethics (Pellegrino, Siegler, & Singer, 1991). We need to get beyond rhetoric to a place where there is true collaboration and consultation among *all* professionals involved in health care.

NOTE

1. According to Meleis (1991), the domain of knowledge is the crux of a discipline such as nursing, and entails practical boundaries (the "current state of investigative interests that emerge from questions that are significant to members of the domain") and theoretical boundaries (the "visionary questions of members") (p. 97). Major concepts within the nursing domain are the nursing client, transitions, interaction, nursing process, environment, nursing therapeutics, and health.

REFERENCES

Allen, D. G. (1992). Feminism, relativism, and the philosophy of science: An overview. In J. L. Thompson, D. G. Allen, & L. Rodrigues-Fisher (Eds.), *Critique, resistance, and action: Working papers in the politics of nursing* (pp. 1-19). New York: National League for Nursing.

Anderson, J. M. (1991). Current directions in nursing research: Toward a poststructuralist and feminist epistemology. *Canadian Journal of Nursing Research, 23*(3), 1-3.

Anderson, J. M., Blue, C., & Lau, A. (1991). Women's perspectives on chronic illness: Ethnicity, ideology and restructuring life. *Social Science and Medicine, 33,* 101-113.

Aroskar, M. (1992). Ethical foundations in nursing for broad health care access. *Scholarly Inquiry for Nursing Practice, 6,* 201-205.

Bridges, J., & Lynam, J. (1993). Informal carers: A Marxist analysis of social, political, and economic forces underpinning the role. *Advances in Nursing Science, 15*(3), 33-48.

Bunting, S. M. (1992). Eve's legacy: An analysis of family caregiving from a feminist perspective. In J. L. Thompson, D. G. Allen, & L. Rodrigues-Fisher (Eds.), *Critique, resistance, and action: Working papers in the politics of nursing* (pp. 53-68). New York: National League for Nursing.

Bunting, S. M., & Campbell, J. C. (1994). Through a feminist lens: A model to guide nursing research. In P. L. Chinn (Ed.), *Advances in methods of inquiry for nursing* (pp. 75-87). Rockville, MD: Aspen.

Butterfield, P. (1990). Thinking upstream: Nurturing a conceptual understanding of the societal context of health behavior. *Advances in Nursing Science, 12*(2), 1-8.

Campbell, J. C., & Bunting, S. (1991). Voices and paradigms: Perspectives on critical and feminist theory in nursing. *Advances in Nursing Science, 13*(3), 1-15.

Chopoorian, T. J. (1986). Reconceptualizing the environment. In P. Moccia (Ed.), *New approaches to theory development* (pp. 39-54). New York: National League for Nursing.

Cooper, M. C. (1988). Covenantal relationships: Grounding for the nursing ethic. *Advances in Nursing Science, 10*(4), 48-59.

Curtin, L. (1993). Health: Reform, refrain or reshuffle? *Nursing Management, 24*(1), 7-8.

Danis, M., & Churchill, L. R. (1991). Autonomy and the common weal. *Hastings Center Report, 21*(1), 25-31.

Donaldson, S. K. (1995). Introduction: Nursing science for nursing practice. In A. Omery, C. E. Kasper, & G. G. Page (Eds.), *In search of nursing science* (pp. 3-12). Thousand Oaks, CA: Sage.

Ericksen, J., Rodney, P., & Starzomski, R. (1995). When is it right to die? *Canadian Nurse, 91*(8), 29-34.

Evans, R. G. (1994). Introduction. In R. G. Evans, M. L. Barer, & T. R. Marmor (Eds.), *Why are some people healthy and others not? The determinants of health of populations* (pp. 3-26). New York: Aldine de Gruyter.

Fagin, C. (1981). Health policy in the nursing curriculum: Why do we need it? *Journal of Advanced Nursing, 6*, 71-73.

Fowler, M. (1990). Social ethics and nursing. In N. L. Chaska (Ed.), *The nursing profession: Turning points* (pp. 24-31). St. Louis, MO: C. V. Mosby.

Fry, S. T. (1985). Individual vs. aggregate good: Ethical tension in nursing practice. *International Journal of Nursing Studies, 22*, 303-310.

Fry, S. T. (1989). Toward a theory of nursing ethics. *Advances in Nursing Science, 11*(4), 9-22.

Fry, S. T. (1992). Neglect of philosophical inquiry in nursing: Cause and effect. In J. F. Kikuchi & H. Simmons (Eds.), *Philosophic inquiry in nursing* (pp. 85-96). Newbury Park, CA: Sage.

Gillis, A. (1992). Allocation of health care resources: The case for health promotion. *Nursing Forum, 27*(4), 21-26.

Hathaway, D., & Strong, M. (1988). Theory, practice and research in transplant nursing. *American Nephrology Nurses Association Journal, 15*(1), 9-12.

Ingersoll, G., Hoffart, N., & Schultz, A. (1990). Health services research in nursing: Current status and future directions. *Nursing Economics, 8*, 229-238.

Jameton, A., & Fowler, M. D. M. (1989). Ethical inquiry and the concept of research. *Advances in Nursing Science, 11*(3), 11-24.

Jennings, B., Callahan, D., & Wolf, S. M. (1987). The professions: Public interest and common good. *Hastings Center Report, 17*(1), 3-10.

Jones, P., & Meleis, A. (1993). Health is empowerment. *Advances in Nursing Science, 15*(3), 1-14.

Kendall, J. (1992). Fighting back: Promoting emancipatory nursing actions. *Advances in Nursing Science, 15*(2), 1-15.

Kjellstrand, C. M. (1992). Disguising unjust rationing by calling it futile therapy. *Bioethics Bulletin, 4*(2), 1-3.

Kleffel, D. (1991a). An ecofeminist analysis of nursing knowledge. *Nursing Forum, 26*(4), 5-18.

Kleffel, D. (1991b). Rethinking the environment as a domain of nursing knowledge. *Advances in Nursing Science, 14*(1), 40-51.

Kornblith, H. (1985). Introduction: What is naturalistic epistemology? In H. Kornblith (Ed.), *Naturalizing epistemology* (pp. 1-13). Cambridge, MA: Bradford.

Kos-Munson, B. A. (1992). Introduction. *Scholarly Inquiry for Nursing Practice, 6*, 179-184.

Kuhn, T. S. (1970). *The structure of scientific revolutions* (2nd ed.). Chicago: University of Chicago Press.

Larsen, J., & Baumgart, A. J. (1992). Overview: Shaping public policy. In A. J. Baumgart & J. Larsen (Eds.), *Canadian nursing faces the future* (2nd ed., pp. 469-492). St. Louis, MO: C. V. Mosby.

Laudan, L. (1977). *Progress and its problems: Toward a theory of scientific growth*. Berkeley: University of California Press.

Lefort, S. (1993). Shaping health policy. *Canadian Nurse, 89*(3), 23-27.

Liaschenko, J. (1993). Feminist ethics and cultural ethos: Revisiting a nursing debate. *Advances in Nursing Science, 15*(4), 71-81.

Luke, C., & Gore, J. (1992). Introduction. In C. Luke & J. Gore (Eds.), *Feminisms and critical pedagogy* (pp. 1-14). New York: Routledge.

May, W. F. (1989). Code, covenant, contract, or philanthropy. In R. M. Veatch (Ed.), *Cross-cultural perspectives in medical ethics: Readings* (pp. 156-173). Boston: Jones & Bartlett.

Meleis, A. I. (1991). *Theoretical nursing: Development and progress* (2nd ed.). Philadelphia: J. B. Lippincott.

Milio, N. (1984). The realities of policy making: Can nurses have an impact? *Journal of Nursing Administration, 14*(3), 18-23.

Moccia, P. (1988). At the fault line: Social activism and caring. *Nursing Outlook, 36*(1), 30-33.

Morreim, E. H. (1988). Cost containment: Challenging fidelity and justice. *Hastings Center Report, 18*(6), 20-25.

Nagelkerk, J., & Henry, B. (1991). Leadership through policy research. *Journal of Nursing Administration, 21*(5), 20-24.

Oberle, K., & Grant, N. (1994). *Results of the AARN initiative regarding the impact of health care cuts*. Unpublished research report, Alberta Association of Registered Nurses, Edmonton.

Pellegrino, E. D., Siegler, M., & Singer, P. A. (1991). Future directions in clinical ethics. *Journal of Clinical Ethics, 2*(1), 5-9.

Penticuff, J. H. (1991). Conceptual issues in nursing ethics research. *Journal of Medicine and Philosophy, 16*, 235-258.

Portnoy, F. L., & Dumas, L. (1994). Nursing for the public good. *Nursing Clinics of North America, 29*, 371-375.

Rachlis, M., & Kushner, C. (1994). *Strong medicine: How to save Canada's health care system*. Toronto: HarperCollins.

Raudonis, B. M., & Griffith, H. (1991). Model for integrating health services research and health care policy formation. *Nursing and Health Care, 12*(1), 32-36.

Reed, P. G. (1989). Nursing theorizing as an ethical endeavor. *Advances in Nursing Science, 11*(3), 1-9.

Reed, P. G. (1995). A treatise on nursing knowledge development for the 21st century: Beyond postmodernism. *Advances in Nursing Science, 17*(3), 70-84.

Rodney, P., & Starzomski, R. (1994). Responding to ethical challenges. *Nursing BC, 26*(2), 10-13.

Sherwin, S. (1992). *No longer patient: Feminist ethics and health care*. Philadelphia: Temple University Press.

Sokolowski, R. (1991). The fiduciary relationship and the nature of professions. In E. D. Pellegrino, R. M. Veatch, & J. P. Langan (Eds.), *Ethics, trust, and the professions: Philosophical and cultural aspects* (pp. 23-43). Washington, DC: Georgetown University Press.

Squires, J. (1993). Introduction. In J. Squires (Ed.), *Principled positions: Postmodernism and the rediscovery of value* (pp. 1-13). London: Lawrence & Wishart.

Stevens, P. (1989). A critical social reconceptualization of environment in nursing: Implications for methodology. *Advances in Nursing Science, 11*(4), 56-68.

Stevens, P. (1992). Who gets care? Access to health care as an arena for nursing action. *Scholarly Inquiry for Nursing Practice, 6*, 185-200.

Storch, J. (1986). In defense of nursing theory. *Canadian Nurse, 82*(1), 16-20.

Thorne, S. E. (1993). *Negotiating health care: The social context of chronic illness.* Newbury Park, CA: Sage.

Watson, S. D. (1994). Minority access and health reform: A civil right to health care. *Journal of Law, Medicine and Ethics, 22*(2), 127-137.

Williams, D. (1991). Health promotion, caring and nursing: Why social activism is necessary. In P. Chinn (Ed.), *Anthology on caring* (pp. 47-58). New York: National League for Nursing.

Yeo, M. (1989). Integration of nursing theory and nursing ethics. *Advances in Nursing Science, 11*(3), 33-42.

Yeo, M. (1993). *Ethics and economics in health care resource allocation.* Ottawa: Queen's University of Ottawa Economic Projects.

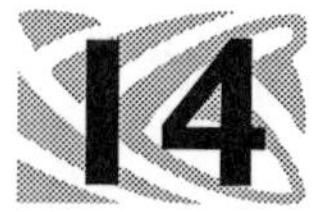

Health Knowledge and the Praxis of Otherness

The Case in the Developing World

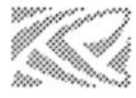

EMÍLIA L. SAPORITI ANGERAMI
FRANCISCO A. CORREIA

In this chapter, we consider the notion of health promotion as a global nursing perspective that emphasizes co-responsibility between people and their societies. We hold the view that many traditional nursing perspectives have inappropriately focused on individuals as the objects of social health efforts rather than subjects with their own attitudes and capability for reciprocity. Health promotion praxis forces us to consider economic interests in health, the context of the human condition, and ecological considerations. Its objectives are the improvement of the quality of life and human dignity, the possibility of offering individuals maximum use of their capacities, and a decent standard of living. True co-responsibility demands a radical revision of established practices and concepts within nursing and health care. We argue that the "praxis of otherness" adds a critical dimension to traditional understanding of the ethical principles by which health care decisions can be enacted. Analyses of the shifting responsibilities within research and health care and of the global context of health and disease, as well as examination of the limitations of traditional ethical perspectives, lead us to a new perspective, one of health as both a right and a duty. Drawing on exemplary issues in developing countries as a source of insight for global interpretations, we introduce in this chapter an exploration of the relationships among social responsibility, ethical thinking, and health promotion.

CO-RESPONSIBILITY

Until the 1960s, health beliefs were located within "assistencialist" parameters, enlightened by the beneficence principle (Correia, 1993). *Beneficence,* from the Latin *bonum facere,* means "to do good," and this is the most ancient principle of medical ethics. The traditional Hippocratic model, which is based upon and oriented to this principle, does not tolerate exceptions to beneficence as long as human beings are suffering or in need of attention and care. "To do good," "do no harm," "take care of health," and "promote quality of life" constitute the maxims of traditional health morality. Until recently, beneficence was of prime importance to medical and nursing conduct. Today, however, it is limited by at least four main factors: the necessity of defining what is good for the patient, the nonacceptance of paternalism and/or maternalism that is embedded in beneficence, the emergence of the criterion of autonomy, and new dimensions of justice in the health arena (Gracia, 1989). In the 1970s, however, many theorists began to look to the principle of autonomy as a means of correcting some of the implications that the beneficence principle created. *Autonomy,* a term derived from the Greek *autós, eu, nomos, lei,* refers to the capacity of the human rational will to make laws for itself. As an ethical principle, autonomy implies the emancipation of human reason, the legislation by the subjects themselves of their lives and attitudes. It orients us toward the capacity of the human person to be and act as subject.

The introduction of the autonomy principle in the health arena provoked a radical change in relationships between health professionals and the recipients of care. Clients of health care now became autonomous subjects wishing to establish interpersonal relations with professionals, sharing health care decisions in partnership and full citizenship rights. Thus health care relationships that had been excessively vertical, monarchic, and sometimes even absolutist were transformed into relationships that were more horizontal, democratic, and symmetrical in character. Although we recognize that there are limits and deficiencies to the application of the autonomy principle, we want to emphasize here that the principle permitted the emergence of the subject in the health arena as someone who deciphers his or her world, who knows how to be an agent, who shows knowledge, and who reveals the mechanisms of health and disease in his or her own vital space.

In the context of the autonomy principle, the role of the researcher has evolved from one of expert who studies populations for their own good to one of participant who acts co-responsibly within a community, articulating knowledge exchange in dynamic interaction with that community. In order to understand how this role can be enacted, it is important to understand a third ethical principle, that of justice. The principle of justice demands that, in additional to being functional and efficient, all attention, all care, and all health systems must be just. It is the principle of justice that obliges us to guarantee the fair, equitable, and universal distribution of the benefits of health services. Over recent years, this principle has emerged as part of conscience citizenship, exemplified by international struggles around articulating health as a right for all people.

The principle of justice directs us toward the optimization of good consequences and acts, including maximum benefit for minimum cost. In application, these obligations impose daunting challenges, such as the problem of quantifying costs and benefits in the absorption of just options for health resources, which are inevitably scarce. For justice to be served, quantification of costs and benefits within societies is imperative. But how do we quantify pain, deficiency, disability, and death? Who is to receive assistance in circumstances in which there are not resources sufficient for all? What will the selection criteria be? It is within this context that we propose the idea of the "praxis of otherness." We consider this an appropriate way to consider global health promotion problems within the complexity of bioethical understanding and particularly within the context of health agency in everyday community life.

THE PRAXIS OF OTHERNESS

Before we specifically address the praxis of otherness, we think it is important to recall its origins in practical philosophy, the reflection about the ethical praxis of individuals and social and political institutions. Several factors are responsible for the development, evolution, and amplification of this practical philosophy. These include recognition that ethics lays the foundation for the criteria and norms required to orient human praxis, recognition of the experience of moral suffering and the outrage provoked by moral abuse, the value that has been ascribed to subjective experience in decision-making processes, and the hermeneutic focus that reestablishes a relationship between the experienced ethos and ethical reflection without falling into the trap of so-called naturalistic fallacy (Viafora, 1990). In addition, there has been serious recognition of the importance of listening to the voice of "the other." For instance, in the context of excessive androcentric rationalism, it has become imperative to listen to women's voices and accept their attitudes about caretaking, attitudes that value compassion and the importance of someone taking care of another. Currently, there is renewed interest in Aristotle's' "political and ethical doctrine," considering "the theoretical and practical crisis of the post-industrial civilization ethical universe" (Viafora, 1990, pp. 22-23). Finally, the contributions of analytic ethics, moral theology, law, and economics have all encouraged and supported the emergence of a practical philosophy of reflection and action (Viafora, 1990). These ideas illustrate the location of our view of the praxis of otherness within practical philosophy.

The preliminary foundation of the notion of "otherness" is the person understood as open, relating, communicating, and intersubjective (Correia, 1993). In the history of philosophy, the notion of the "other" is not new. In various discussions, it has been ascribed different meanings: to be an other, to belong to the other, the problem of the other, characteristic of what belongs to the other, acknowledging the other, and so forth. From the time of Aristotle, the "other" has been an important concept in the understanding of human relations and their implications.

According to Vaz (1968), Hegel reestablished the "problem of the other" in his work *Phenomenology of the Spirit* and influenced subsequent schools of thought such as existentialism, Marxism, phenomenology, and personalism. The philosophers Kierkegaard, Husserl, and Scheler (the "classics" of "other" philosophy), and Hartmann, Mounier, Madinier, Lacroix, Malverne, Heidegger, Jaspers, Marcel, Sartre, and Levinas have all treated the theme of "other" in their own ways. However, in the recent history of ethics, "otherness" has often been veiled in the notion of "person," and all consequences for ethical action have not been extracted from it. It was Laín Entralgo (1961, 1983) who initiated exploration of this theme in the doctor-patient relationship and Dussel (1972, 1986) who introduced it to the context of liberation ethics in Latin America. We owe our conception of otherness to them: Laín Entralgo (1983) positions the notion of otherness in the health arena, and Dussel (1986) expresses otherness in the context of the Third World.

We present the praxis of otherness in health promotion and research because it not only fills some gaps and limitations provoked by the principles of beneficence, autonomy, and justice, it also transcends them. We find that otherness permits us not only to trace a conductive thread of reflection, but to consider thematically all of bioethics. Further, we believe it meets the present ethical demands that the person be viewed as subject, protagonist, and critical user, free to be responsible for health services; it gives moral competence back to the individual. In addition, we believe it sensitizes us to acknowledge ethical problems within the scope of life and health in a reciprocal manner (the "other" is also "myself") because it means common sympathy and reciprocal responsibility. From our perspective, adopting a praxis of otherness evokes a transformational criterion within relationships. It is no longer a rationalist model of man, according to which the professional/researcher confuses motive maturation with indifference to nature and the environment, humanity, and the realities of the impoverished, marginalized, excluded majority. The praxis of otherness ruptures our alignment with paternalism and/or maternalism, assistencialism, functionalism, and absolutism and allows exchange or permutation of knowledge in participative and co-responsible interaction. It allows, therefore, a relationship of collaboration between adult, mutually respectful parties in health care (client and health care provider). Finally, it is our view that a praxis of otherness permits a kind of consensus that is difficult within the varied anthropological and value systems of pluralistic societies.

In proposing the praxis of otherness, we want to establish the person as the foundation of all reflection and of all bioethical practice—not the person enclosed in him- or herself, but the person conceived as open and related, engaged reciprocally with another person or other persons (in the sense of the needy, excluded multitude). Otherness, therefore, permits us not only to lay a foundation for but also to structure and articulate the contents of bioethics. Under the light of otherness, one can break from the "totality" that disguises or alienates the other (person, community, or multitude). The principle unveils the other and makes her or him burst forth as something different from what she or he is within the social system. The other exists and acts, not because she or he merely fights to survive, is unhealthy, does not have resources to meet her or his basic needs (food, shelter, education, and so on), dies precociously, or has insufficient health care. No, the other is equal, autonomous, and co-responsible.

CONTEXTUALIZING HEALTH AND DISEASE

The concepts of health and disease change according to the circumstances of time and place. Social and political changes, as well as scientific and technological advances, contribute to successive redefinition. The international proposals for primary health care agreed upon in the Alma-Ata Charter (World Health Organization, 1978) constitute a broad conception of strategies to reorient resources within the health care sector to meet the needs of societies worldwide. In countries where the health care system has been successfully reformulated, primary care and sanitation are initial steps in which problems of minor technical, diagnostic, and therapeutic difficulty are solved, and those of greater complexity are considered secondary. Unfortunately, this conceptualization often clashes with political aims. In underdeveloped countries where an organized and articulated, regionalized health care delivery system is not yet possible, primary care receives a kind of selective attention, aiming at marginalized populations who live on the periphery of cities or in rural areas. The outcome of such programs is the use of personnel with low qualifications trained in the use of simple technologies, able to access complex or sophisticated resources only with difficulty. Under such conditions, it is impossible to maintain the quality of services at necessary levels (Testa, 1992).

Facing this reality, health reform in several countries has become part of a broad social and political restructuring process within an overall social transformation movement. Health ceases to be considered an abstract concept and becomes a human right. It is no longer a personal problem, but a matter of state. The state becomes responsible for formulating health programs and for determining the major normative instruments to care delivery. Such a politically determined health-disease concept becomes central to the definition of population problems and strategies. Mainetti (1990) articulates this as a third generation of rights, beyond basic ecological questions and toward rights to peace and development, as well as the respect for common patrimony and future generations. He explains how transition from the status of right to health toward one of justice is established: Health surpasses the question of individual rights (such as sanitary assistance) and, in direct contrast to threatened lives, assumes the dimension of a just macrobioethics (the population explosion, ecological and nuclear catastrophes), which includes accountability for the rights of future generations. Such a view looks into the future, reflecting about the values of the biological revolution, of bioengineering, of environmental and antinuclear bioethics, of epidemiological transition, and of the directives of preventive, educative, and health promotion actions.

In the Ottawa Charter (World Health Organization, 1986), the fundamental conditions and resources for health are expressed as peace, shelter, education, food, income, a stable ecosystem, sustainable resources, social justice, and equity. The charter claims that improvement in health requires a secure foundation in the basic prerequisites. These concepts reveal a deep transformation in health paradigms, evidence that the traditional ways of planning and intervening in health have been untenable because they were restricted to the assistencialist and/or functionalist models, in turn guided by the beneficence principle. In the process of health redemocratization, particularly in the countries where resources are scarce and distribution quantity and quality are unequal, "coparticipation" has emerged as a powerful idea. It represents a space where the population acknowledges ownership of a service and reflects a compromise in which mutual commitment of responsibility for health is established. It is on this social participation that democratic relationships are built.

Particularly in countries where political and social rights have been developed under authoritarian models, the concept of citizenship becomes important. Attainment of full citizenship is a process under construction, and the right to health becomes part of a new order established between the rights of the citizen and the duties of the state. This new worldwide order demands that the political-social spheres of citizenship are enlarged until a worldwide citizenship emerges and citizens become historicized and informed. Health education becomes part of the transition from regulated citizenship based on compensatory health policies to full citizenship that recognizes equal rights for all as far as health is concerned.

Exercising the praxis of otherness starts with the reflections of professionals who are interested in more just systems and who are prepared to act within defined territories. To comprehend the construction of such praxis, one must have an opportunity to understand current thinking and examine possibilities, because it is within a political-operative space that an interactive population service occurs. That is, it is possible to visualize a specific population living in a particular time and space, with its own health problems, and interacting with distinctive service-providing units, and to come to appreciate strategies that are currently in practice. The example we offer is an observation of a basic health unit in Brazil, understood as a subsystem of the health system or, in the Brazilian case, a minor part of health care delivery (Mendes, 1994). This example illustrates, using a concrete situation, the relationships that are established among government politics, environment and development, service organization, and health practices.

The health care unit is located in a small community with a population of 8,800 inhabitants. It is 10 kilometers from Ribeirão Preto, Brazil, a city of 457,037 people, which serves as a point of reference. As Ribeirão Preto is an important industrial agricultural center, it has a high per capita income and the population's standard of living is considered superior to that of other regions. Because Brazil is so geographically vast and regionalized, with diverse development situations and health problems specific to each region, it is impossible to generalize about the country as a whole. Some 30 years ago, this exemplary small community was composed of an essentially rural population and the village supported its survival by producing agricultural goods for local markets: coffee, cereals, cotton, and others. In terms of health care, there was a child care unit and another unit to assist trachoma patients. Persons with other diseases were referred to city hospitals. Guided by the beneficence model, clinic and hospital visits were free. Then changes occurred: The petroleum crisis in the 1970s changed the Ribeirão Preto region from a coffee-producing area to one of the greatest producers of alcohol, a renewable alternative energy source. The pro-alcohol project brought unionization to the population, causing deep transformations in the rural areas and subsequently the urban areas. The rural population left the farms for the cities, creating belts of poverty around them and generating problems associated with basic sanitation, shelter, violence, and constant migration. Although the pro-alcohol project brought development and a desirable solution to energy needs in the region, the social and health problems it created are far from being resolved, even today.

Today, the community has a more diverse population than it had 30 years ago. It has urban characteristics, and most of the inhabitants have temporary jobs in agriculture or in the cities. Newcomers were attracted to housing complexes constructed by the government, though these have provoked conflicts with former residents who have been negatively affected by the changes in their area. This rural zone was transformed to produce a single agricultural crop, sugarcane, managed in a system of land leasing to large alcohol and sugar mills, which incorporate a workforce that comes from the cities to complete a day's work or lives in lodgings constructed for migrants. The utilization of a large labor force composed primarily of children and women to cut the sugarcane has created serious health and education problems; workers are illiterate and poor, having abandoned their homes and schools. Because this kind of work is seasonal and migratory, men come from other regions of the country, abandoning their wives and children. Female workers are also responsible for housework and child care, besides their active participation in cutting sugarcane, with consequent negative outcomes on their physical and mental health. The question of whether development can occur without institutionalized birth control is still a political polemic. The ethical and social aspects of this fundamental question must be considered if there are to be concrete solutions that respect the individuality of families (Szmhrecsanyi, 1988).

The living conditions of this population in the cities reflect extreme poverty; people live in unhealthy houses without basic sanitation, garbage collection, or water, and there are frequent accidents owing to inadequate transportation to and from the work sites in the fields (Oliveira & Oliveira, 1981). The diseases found among the members of this workforce are related to the use of agrotoxics, snakebites, trauma with sharp instruments, skin and respiratory diseases, malnutrition, posture problems, and diseases affecting physical and psychological development. Thus a polarity is created: on the one hand, humans damaging the environment; on the other, the environment attacking humans.

Within the Brazilian health care system, the basic health unit has progressively enlarged its coverage in this region, and now operates 24 hours per day. The health team is composed of general practitioners and some specialists, dentists, nurses, auxiliary personnel, and administrative personnel. Care is oriented toward both children and adults (with a special program for women) and includes dental treatment and nursing activities. Nurses are in charge of the coordination and execution of vaccination programs, orientation before and after medical consultations, and emergency attention for respiratory crises and accidents. They perform community work, including home visits, epidemiological supervision, and support in an institution for preschool children and a home for aged women. Severely ill patients are referred to the city hospital. The epidemiological profile includes diarrhea, hypertension, diabetes mellitus, respiratory and skin diseases, and work-related accidents, especially trauma and ocular lesions. Tuberculosis and Hansen's disease (leprosy) are rare. The HIV/AIDS program is centralized, and the sick are referred to more advanced units. Service is clearly aimed at quick response to clients' health problems in reaction to specific demands.

Overcoming poverty and inequalities must be part of the conscientization process of a people. As Freire (1990) states, it is necessary to transform the naive conscience of critical persons within a society, so that they claim their rights and demand worthy living conditions. In our interviews with members of this health care team, we noted reservations about participatory processes in health care, as some perceived that they might lose their mechanisms of leadership and control. Although poorly organized, members of the population are capable of reporting their problems and are determined to fight for their rights. We therefore understand this to be a conflict in which negotiations have not yet succeeded in releasing the critical and creative capacities of those involved.

HEALTH: RIGHT AND DUTY

The example presented above reveals health as a result of multiple determinants, including food, income, environment, education, work, leisure, freedom, and access to health resources. Various forms of social organization and access to production can generate great inequities within health. In spite of the efforts of the World Health Organization and of the Pan-American Health Organization to extend the right of health to the populations of all nations, it is possible to identify a number of challenges that remain in developing countries, including Brazil.

The right to health means a guarantee by the state of a worthy standard of living, universal and equal access to health promotion, protection and recovery of health, and the possibility of full development as a human being. It is evident that actualization of this ideology depends on the state's formulation of explicit policies, allowing the population to control administrative processes as well as to evaluate established social and economic priorities. From this broad concept of health emerges the notion of health as a right, where the limitations and obstacles are of a structural nature and must be removed through social organization.

Nogueira (1994) describes a diversity of processes by which the users of health services submit to the rhythm of health care attitudes to produce only the effects the service providers expect. Because clients are expected to fit into the logic of the service organization, they are obliged to search within specialties and subspecialties to obtain portions of interventions for parts of their bodies, passively receive information, follow orders, and collaborate in what others determine is good for them. In nursing work, this constitutes care plans that assign fragmented tasks to auxiliary personnel with low qualifications. This system of providing care, with its rigid scheme of control and centralized supervision, has been severely criticized for its incompatibility with a commitment to co-responsibility on the part of the health worker.

An organizational model such as this creates difficulties for the introduction of new concepts of participative administration within the health team, in which ancient training strategies are replaced by human resources policies that capitalize on human organizational potential. Gracia (1990a) argues that one of the new notions introduced in the health arena is the concept of right, which has been expressed in the rights of patients, in the individual view, and in the egalitarian and unanimous rights of all citizens. Economy and health are two opposing forces when the high cost of services and the low resoluteness of individuals' actions are considered.

In considering this problem, Mainetti (1990) shows its amplitude. When health is considered a consumer good within a population that is increasingly more chronic and aged, health services show the radical economic implications: more expensive medical services as a consequence of high technology, bad praxis and abuse of social security, and excessive specialization, among others. Such changes lead to excesses in consumption and expenses and to scarcity of available resources, and impose a system of so-called rational designation. Financing health care reform becomes the nucleus of sanitation politics, which in turn becomes an important political component of the "doing good" state. It is no longer possible to generate resources outside the context of a strategic planning process that articulates population interests in a better standard of living, especially for those in great need. Discussions aimed at obtaining more resources for the health sector and more equitable social distribution lead to analysis of inefficiencies of services and consequent dissatisfaction for both users and health workers.

Inefficiency and waste in the health sector are considered a worldwide problem. Inefficiency results from the spending of more resources than necessary to achieve particular outcomes, and waste is the irresponsible or poor use of resources. The common result is failure to obtain expected improvement in the health status of the population. For example, sources of waste arise from political decisions on the part of authorities at the administrative level assigning tasks to health agents that do not fit sanitation priorities (Parker & Newbrander, 1994). In order to reduce this problem, guidelines and priorities must be established according to ethical principles. Decisions must follow debate and consensus. The formulation of objectives, principles, and criteria is a conjoint responsibility of those who are responsible for service administration and all actual and potential health service recipients. Openness and transparency are moral requisites indispensable to the organizations exerting power and to the individuals representing them.

In this context, Lonning (1994) states that the best way to judge a health system from a moral point of view is to consider whether it enhances or reduces inequities between the rich and the poor as far as access to public services is concerned. When scarce resources are wasted due to inefficiency, the most disadvantaged are inevitably those who most need the services.

Demand for high-quality services emerges when the client has an improved economic and cultural context. The poorest are often so removed from access that they have no basis upon which to complain about the little they receive (Gracia, 1990b). In introducing the autonomy issue, bioethical theory has made a valuable contribution to the basic conditions of citizenship. Patients and their families assume the right to decide about health practices and to participate in the diagnostic and treatment process. The notion of quality of service assumes that the caregiver has pride in the service provided and that the client has the right to express opinions and choose among alternative procedures with full knowledge of associated risks, and is ready to collaborate with the processes of diagnosis and treatment. Although the concept of the client's role in quality of service is recent, it is fundamental for achieving health care reform goals as expressed by rights and duties. Citizens now organize themselves and insist that the taxes they pay be utilized with maximum efficiency.

However, notions of right and duty are not enough if we do not also add the intention to recover, in the developed and developing worlds, the notion of virtues, a set of human qualities to be developed by professionals and that can be understood as sensitivity—sensitivity to pain, suffering, and the needs of others such as multiple or ethnic and cultural minorities. In our view, interdisciplinary and intercultural work contributes strongly to that sensitivity, and should be considered a necessary task in every local institution, not only in the sense of theoretical and technological actions, but in the sense of resources that permit attention to health to reach a level compatible with the need for health. As far as health is concerned in developing countries, islands of high technology are surrounded by populations greatly in need of basic health resources. Extreme situations occur when a few have access to everything and use a significant proportion of the available resources while many are deprived of even the simplest services, with the aggravating circumstance that they do not even know their right to health or how to exert it. Such disparity is far from being solved and will require mutual collaboration between the countries that generate the latest knowledge and technology and those that still strive for justice and a fair quality of life. Health promotion praxis therefore requires the practice of justice and full citizenship among all peoples. Only in that way will we reach peace and health for all.

CONCLUSION

What is the role of clinicians and researchers in enacting the praxis of otherness? Introducing a participative model into the community (understood as any local area in which health actions are practiced) creates an educative and preventive influence that can generate intervention projects. Discussion of research results or program options gradually exerts a transforming influence upon the community. In this way, co-responsibility between professionals and the community is developed and exercised in a dynamic and permanent manner, allowing priorities and problems to emerge from and be addressed within the community's experienced reality.

This idealistic view is still far from the usual practice in providing assistance in most of the developing world, or in conducting research. The guidelines derived from social politics are highly bureaucratized, rooted in the beneficence model, in the utilitarian philosophy, and in the belief in maximum production with minimum cost. There is failure to consider the needs of the user. Health professionals have not incorporated the new concepts of health and bioethics into their work. They continue to consider themselves the holders of power and knowledge, negating the population's right to make health decisions and maintain cultural traditions.

The training of health promotion researchers according to normative models instills deep understanding in specific topics and methods and sensitivity to familiar means of knowledge production. Yet what both health practitioners and scientists require to work in developing countries is a genuine commitment to the communities in which they are working. The growing number of cooperative international projects investigating health and health assistance, if adequately performed, represent a potential source of health knowledge not only to the sponsoring countries but also to the recipient ones. Professionals' and nations' revision of current ideas of the praxis of otherness is an urgent concern, for when the dominant country establishes strategies and goals, project results will not meet the aspirations of countries with fewer resources, and aid and research may become expropriated into domination politics.

In contrast to the polemic created by partnership development projects in which foreign investigators with particular worldviews study people of different cultures, we believe that it is possible to familiarize investigators with cultural differences so that their projects can be adapted as needed. This practice requires that foreign and national investigators cooperate in every phase of a project. Thus co-responsibility is practiced not only in scientific and ethical terms, but also in efforts toward the achievement of specific objectives. The closer the cooperation, the more efficacious the communication and the more respect there will be among individual citizens, peoples, lawmakers, and authorities. The process of collaboration is therefore a path that can reduce distances between developed and developing countries, and thus can benefit both. The continuous domination by rich countries of the poor through expropriation and excessive economic growth harms the environment and endangers the health of human beings. Through the revision of established practices and the exercise of shared responsibility among government and nongovernment organizations and individual citizens, health promotion can be enacted globally through the praxis of otherness.

REFERENCES

Correia, F. A. (1993). *A alteridade como critério fundamental e englobante da bioética* [Otherness as a global and fundamental criterion of bioethics]. Unpublished doctoral thesis, Universidade de Campinas, Campinas, Brazil.

Dussel, E. (1972). *Para una destruccion de la história de la ética* [For a destruction of the history of ethics]. Mendoza, Argentina: Ser y Tiempo.

Dussel, E. (1986). *Ética comunitária* [Community ethics]. Petrópolis, Brazil: Editora Vozes.

Freire, P. (1990). *Educação como prática da liberdade* [Education as a form of freedom] (10th ed.). São Paulo: Paz e Terra.

Gracia, D. (1989). *Fundamentos de bioética* [Foundations of bioethics]. Madrid: EUDEMA.

Gracia, D. (1990a). Introduction: Medical bioethics. *Bulletin of the Pan American Health Organization, 24,* 355-360.

Gracia, D. (1990b). What constitutes a just health services system and should scarce resources be allocated? *Bulletin of the Pan American Health Organization, 24,* 550-565.

Laín Entralgo, P. (1961). *Teoria y realidad del otro* [Theory and reality of the other]. Madrid: Revista del Ocidente.

Laín Entralgo, P. (1983). *La relación médico-enfermo* [The physician-patient relationship]. Madrid: Alianza Editorial.

Lonning, I. (1994). Ethical aspects of wastage. *World Health Forum, 15*(2), 125-126.

Mainetti, J. A. (1990). Bioethics: A new health philosophy. *Bulletin of the Pan American Health Organization, 24,* 578-581.

Mendes, E. V. (Ed.). (1994). *Distrito sanitário: O processo social de mudança das práticas sanitárias do Sistema Unico de Saúde* [Health center: The process of change in practices in the health system] (2nd ed.). São Paulo/Rio de Janeiro: Hucitec/ABRASCO.

Nogueira, R. P. (1994). *Perspectivas da qualidade em saúde* [Perspectives of quality in health]. Rio de Janeiro: Qualitymark.

Oliveira, J. E. D., & Oliveira, M. H. S. P. (Eds.). (1981). *"Boias frias": Uma realidade brasileira* ["Farmworkers": A Brazilian reality]. São Paulo: CNPq/Acadêmia de Ciências do Estado de São Paulo.

Parker, D., & Newbrander, W. (1994). Tackling wastage and inefficiency in the health sector. *World Health Forum, 15*(2), 107-126.

Szmhrecsanyi, M. I. (1988). *Educação e fecundidade: Ideologia, teoria, e método na sociologia da reprodução humana* [Education and fertility: Ideology, theory, and method in the sociology of human fertility]. São Paulo: Hucitec/EDUSP.

Testa, M. (1992). *Pensar em saúde* [Thinking in health]. Pôrto Alegre, Brazil: Artes Médicas.

Vaz, M. C. de L. (1968). *Ontologia e história* [Ontology and history]. São Paulo: Duas Cidades.

Viafora, C. (1990). *Vent'anmi di bioética: Idee, protagonisti, istituzioni* [Twenty years of bioethics: Ideas, leading people, institutions]. Padua/Rome: Fondazione Lanza/ Gregoriana Libreria Editrice.

World Health Organization. (1978). The Alma Ata Conference on Primary Health Care. *WHO Chronicle, 32*, 409-430.

World Health Organization. (1986, November). Ottawa Charter for Health Promotion. In World Health Organization, *Proceedings of the International Conference on Health Promotion.* Ottawa: World Health Organization/Health and Welfare Canada/Canadian Public Health Association.

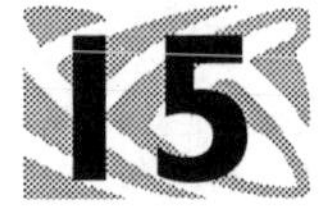

Action Research as Authentic Methodology for the Study of Nursing

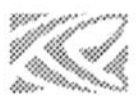

SANDRA RASMUSSEN

Nursing is failing to fulfill its social contract because it follows alien methodology. Methodology is the way nurses care for clients, conduct research, and construct theory. Alien methodology jeopardizes practice, confounds theory, and threatens the very essence of nursing itself. In contrast, authentic methodology affirms and advances the scientific, practical, and ethical tenets of nursing.

In 1979, Margaret Newman suggested action research as a method for developing *theories of practice* for nursing. Action research is a participatory process by which the nurse and client collaborate to effect change and generate knowledge about a particular health problem. The attributes of action research include mutuality, participation, and systematic inquiry; immediacy, relevance, and usefulness; and action, skill development, and learning. All participants benefit directly from action research. In this chapter, I propose action research as authentic methodology for the study of nursing.

I begin by underscoring the tenets of contemporary nursing and then explain what I mean by *alien* and *authentic methodology.* I will then chronicle the origins and development of action research and illustrate how the social philosophy of Jürgen Habermas, especially his theory of communicative action, supports and strengthens action research for nursing. I will also show how nurses engaged in action research are making a major contribution to nursing's fulfillment of its social contract, and then conclude the chapter with a short commentary on the politics of method.

THE NATURE OF NURSING

Authentic methodology affirms and advances the tenets of nursing. Yet what are the tenets of nursing today? Nursing is a scientific holistic process directed toward personal and public well-being. In form, nursing is a scientific profession with a specific knowledge base in the arts, sciences, and nursing. Its practice is governed by legal definitions and regulations and guided by professional standards and a code of ethics. In substance, nursing is a holistic process directed toward well-being. Three concepts characterize contemporary nursing: holism, process, and well-being.

- Client, nurse, and environment constitute a collaborative *whole.*
- *Process* is a systematic series of interdependent actions directed toward a goal.
- *Well-being* is maximum human functioning.

In current usage, the term *client* includes individual, group, and community. In this context, environment is an active variable, not merely the context in which the nurse and client collaborate. Environment includes the context, the ecology, and the social and cultural conditions that influence client and nurse.

THE QUEST FOR METHODOLOGY

Methodology may be defined as a way, technique, or process of or for doing something. The term comes from the Greek word *methodos,* which means "way," a way followed, the pursuit of a path. Methodology is the way nurses know and do nursing.

Alien Methodology

Traditionally, nurses have borrowed or shared methodology. However, as Stevens (1984) points out, "rigorous adherence to borrowed methods is just as likely to retard the development of nursing as is the adherence to borrowed subject matter. The methods that work for one discipline may not for another" (p. 205). Borrowed or shared methodology is not alien simply because it is borrowed or shared, but because it is contrary to nursing.

For the first 75 years of the twentieth century, nursing relied on the empirical-analytic approach, classic experimental design, and quantitative analysis, which produced much technical knowledge. Newman (1979) notes that "just as social scientists have recognized that the methods of physical science could not totally satisfy their needs, so also nursing scientists are discovering that the methods of traditional science may not be sufficient for their needs" (p. 69). Empiricism and quantitative methodology are not per se faulty. Yet, given the holistic nature of contemporary nursing, I question whether an empirical-analytic, quantitative approach should continue as the primary methodology of nursing.

In the mid-1970s, nurses and other social scientists began to employ more qualitative methods. Many nurses who embraced an organismic worldview found existentialism and phenomenology to be sound philosophy for nursing theory. Qualitative methodology was an appealing alternative to the empirical-analytic approach, with its rigorous reliance on measurement. Qualitative methodology seems to "fit" well with the evolving theories of nursing. Unfortunately, the current health care environment, with its demands for hard data, seems especially hostile toward qualitative methodology.

Any methodology employed by nurses to know and do nursing that violates the nature of nursing can be considered alien. As nursing evolves as a profession, methodology that once supported nursing may be unsound, even false today.

Authentic Methodology

If, then, nursing is a scientific holistic process directed toward personal and public well-being, what is authentic methodology for nursing? Authentic methodology affirms and advances the scientific, practical, and ethical tenets of nursing. For several decades, nurses have been calling for methodology to match the phenomenon under inquiry. Stevens (1984) argues that reliance on the hard sciences and classic experimental design ignores the major realities of nursing phenomena. She does not offer a solution to this methodological problem, but she issues a challenge: "It seems evident that nursing, with its complexity of subject matter, must develop unique methods of inquiry if it is to acquire meaningful knowledge. Creative methodology, based on the nature of the phenomenon under inquiry, is called for, rather than narrow adherence to the methods of a different discipline" (p. 208).

"Searching for More Holistic Methods of Inquiry" is the title of the last chapter of Newman's 1979 book *Theory Development in Nursing.* In that volume, Newman questions whether or not the phenomena being measured in much of nursing research are really manifestations of wholeness. "As nursing scientists become increasingly sophisticated in methodology and confident in the focus of nursing inquiry," she writes, "there is a need to develop methods which will depict the holistic, dynamic nature of man as a living system in a constantly changing world" (p. 69). Newman suggests *action research* as a method for developing theories of practice for nursing. In 1990, Newman again sounded a clarion call for methodology consistent with the philosophical and theoretical perspective of the discipline.

Holter (1988) has written of a gap between nursing practice and nursing theory. She questions the adequacy of both empiricism and phenomenology as appropriate foundations for nursing. Neither philosophical approach supports the holistic nature ascribed to nursing today. Holter proposes *critical theory,* as propounded by Jürgen Habermas, as a theoretical foundation for the development of nursing, because of its holistic orientation.

ACTION RESEARCH: ORIGINS AND DEVELOPMENT

Origins: 1940s

During and immediately after World War II, many psychologists, sociologists, anthropologists, and psychiatrists in Great Britain and the United States engaged in problem-centered research. This pragmatic interest reflected the desire for social science to reach a level of practical usefulness commensurate with social needs. Institutes and research centers developed to support these action programs.

Studies, reports, and publications were legion. Client systems varied widely: organizations, industry, culture, community, small groups, and individuals. Yet the approaches were similar: action research. Scientists and clients collaborated to effect change and develop knowledge about particular social problems.

Several social scientists associate the term *action research* with Kurt Lewin (1946), who conceived of action research as a "spiral of steps each of which is composed of a circle of planning, action, and fact-finding" (p. 38). In subsequent years, social scientists employed, extended, and expanded Lewin's basic work. However, his emphasis on participatory collaboration between client and researcher remained central.

Retrenchment: 1950s

Following World War II, and particularly during the 1950s in the United States, social scientists separated themselves from the practical world. Academic departmentalism returned and further increased the gap between theory and practice. Federal bureaucracies, which controlled much funding, institutionalized the split by funding discovery first and then, if at all, application.

Awakening: 1960s, 1970s

In the United States in the 1960s and 1970s, the civil rights movement, the Vietnam War, and the Great Society programs of the

1960s awakened social concerns that transcended disciplines. "Think globally, act locally" became a rallying cry for community coalitions and community action.

Public policy emerged as an element, course, or concentration at many colleges and universities. Graduate programs such as the social-clinical psychology program at the Wright Institute in California tried to break down traditional barriers between research and action. The faculties of arts and sciences, medicine, education, and divinity at Harvard developed a joint doctoral program in clinical psychology and public practice.

International scholars debated the scientific merits and practical value of action research, for example, the presentations by Orlando Fals Borda, Ulf Himmelstrand, and Paul Ocquist at the Symposium on Action Research and Scientific Analysis in Cartagena, Colombia, in 1977. According to Ocquist (1978), "Pragmatism and Dialectical Materialism conceptualize the union of theory and practice. Both consider that the function of scientific ideas or theory is to guide action or practice. Action or practice in turn must be guided by ideas or theory or they are meaningless" (pp. 160-161). In essence, theory without action is meaningless.

Organizations began to use action research to generate knowledge for problem solving. Susman and Evered (1978), who are organizational scientists, viewed action research as a cyclical process with five phases: diagnosing, action planning, action taking, evaluating, and specifying learning. Collaboration between the client system and the action researcher determined each phase of the action research process.

Resurgence: 1980s to Present

Beginning in the 1980s, increasing numbers of nurses and other social scientists discovered critical theory as a ground for action research. Critical theory owes its origins to Hegel and Marx; its twentieth-century systematization to Horkheimer, Adorno, and their associates at the Institute for Social Research in Frankfurt; and its present-day development to Habermas and his colleagues. Horkheimer recognized that reason alone had become an instrument of domination and control. For Horkheimer, writing in 1937, the thinker must relate all theories to practical attitudes and the social strata that they reflect. Critical theory linked theory with praxis. When thought was linked to social justice, thought could be emancipatory. And it was critical theory that addressed the political oppression of his day (see Horkheimer, 1972).

THE SOCIAL PHILOSOPHY OF JÜRGEN HABERMAS

Communicative Action

Habermas decried the rift between the theoretical and practical caused by modern science. With the rise of modern science, theory became logically integrated systems of quantitative observations and measurements. The practical was absorbed into the sphere of the technical. The well-being of the *polis* became a technical-administrative problem. Habermas argued that even a civilization that has been rendered scientific is not granted dispensation from practical questions. Accepting this challenge, Habermas moved forward to develop a postpositivist methodology of social inquiry. Through a rigorous process of reconstructive science, Habermas grounded social theory somewhere "between philosophy and science."

Habermas set forth his theory of society in his masterwork *The Theory of Communicative Action* (1984, 1987). Three interrelated objectives guided the work: (a) to develop a concept of communicative rationality that is no longer based on the subjectivist and individualist foundations of modern social and political theory; (b) to construct a concept of society that integrates the lifeworld and system paradigms, an integrating of views from "inside and outside"; and (c) to propose a critical theory of modern life that accounts for its tensions, distortions, and pathologies in a way that suggests a redirection rather than an abandonment of the project of enlightenment.

Communicative action is the collaborative dynamic by which participants come to *understanding* with one another. Communicative action is action oriented to mutual understanding. Based on mutual understanding, participants are able to coordinate their actions to initiate *goal setting* and *goal-directed action*. United through mutual understanding, participants act to construct the shared representations, norms, and expectations that hold societies together.

How does Habermas's theory of communicative action support and direct action research for nursing? Communicative action as articulated by Habermas is the dynamic by which client, nurse, and environment come to understand one another. Based on mutual understanding, client, nurse, and environment collaborate (coordinate their actions) and move toward a goal of well-being. Communicative action determines each step of the process: assessment, diagnosis, planning, action, evaluation, and learning. Change in well-being (practical) and knowledge about well-being (theoretical) occur.

Validity

How valid is action research as methodology for nursing? Habermas's theory of communicative action and law helps answer this question (see especially Deflem, 1996). Habermas makes the case that for law to be valid it must derive its legitimacy from those to whom it is applied. Valid law is derived from a process of mutual understanding (communicative rationality). Law cannot be legitimated on the basis of strategic power alone (cognitive-instrumental rationality). Communication is central for the production of legitimate law.

Nursing is valid when it derives its legitimacy from those to whom it is applied, that is, clients. Communication is central to the production of legitimate nursing. As stated, communicative action is the dynamic by which client, nurse, and environment come to understand one another. Communicative action determines each step of the action research process.

Social Relevance

What is the social relevance of action research for nursing? Habermas asserts that discourse at the level of communicative action is *emancipatory*. For Habermas, discourse ethics contains two substantial moral principles, justice and solidarity. *Justice* refers to equal respect and equal rights for all; *solidarity* refers to empathy and care for the well-being of our fellow human beings.

Not all action research is guided by critical theory and its emancipatory interests. However, given the nature of current health care issues, the pursuit of emancipatory interests is important for nursing. Action research for nursing can be emancipatory; justice and solidarity characterize this emancipation.

ACTION RESEARCH FOR NURSING

Today, many diverse disciplines employ action research: social scientists and public officials, corporate managers and human rights advocates, educators and nurses. Nurses engaged in action research are making major contributions to nursing.

Action research increases clinical efficacy. Jillings (1992) used participatory action research in the context of cardiac rehabilitation. Within a repeated focus group format, clients became active collaborators; they defined issues, specified recommendations, and developed directives. Norman and Brandeis (1992) addressed the needs of cancer survivors; they employed an action research approach involving survivors themselves, nurses, other members of the medical team, and administrators to develop programs and overcome service barriers. Fact-finding, planning, action, and evaluation served as a basis for structuring objectives and action; research results guided planning and theory development. The Nottingham Mothers' Stop Smoking Project, an action research project, was extremely successful in helping women stop smoking during pregnancy and in reinforcing nonsmoking behavior (Power, Gillies, Madeley, & Abbott, 1989).

Action research strengthens studies of the quality of care. Patton (1993) reports that action research guided continual quality improvement in a cancer center. Laitinen (1994) describes an ongoing action research project to evaluate quality of care from the point of view of both patients and their informal caregivers. Nurses have noted the affinity between action research and quality circles. In several studies, action research has reflected the quality of care conceptual framework of structure, process, and outcome. Developed by Fetterman (1995) and associates, empowerment evaluation builds on action research, community psychology, and action anthropology. It is an open, democratic, group process that involves the people affected by the evaluation. Members of the group are responsible for every strategy of the evaluation, from planning to reporting findings and recommendations.

Action research encourages change initiatives. It has long been recognized as an approach for planned change within organizations. Moch, Roth, Pederson, Groh-Demers, and Siler (1994) developed an action research plan to promote a healthier work environment. Ditson (1994) conducted an action research project that identified and reduced high turnover rates of homemakers and home health aides. Degerhammar and Wade (1991) used a Lewinian framework to introduce a new system of care delivery into a surgical ward. Titchen and Binnie (1993) employed action research to develop patient-centered nursing in an acute medical unit. Using action research in the form of a quasi-experimental time-series study, Armitage, Chapney-Smith, and Andrews (1991) implemented primary nursing in two long-term psychiatric wards.

Action research fosters student learning in contemporary nursing. Employing action research, Jasper (1994) implemented student-centered learning; Donaldson (1992) developed learning contracts. McCaugherty (1991a, 1991b) developed a teaching model to help students integrate theory and practice to bridge the theory-practice gap.

Action research affords nurses authentic methodology for scholarly study. It has provided the theory base for many scholarly presentations and doctoral dissertations by nurses (Jillings, 1992; Rasmussen, 1984, 1992, 1994; Waldow, 1992; Watts, 1991). Finally, action research expedites emancipation (for an example, see Waldow, 1992).

THE POLITICS OF METHOD

Today, social scientists recognize participatory action research and action science as forms of action research. This diversity is confusing for some nurses and social scientists. In the early development of nursing theory, Stevens (1984) asked nurses to suspend the urge to define terms precisely and to accept more global formulations. In our search for meaningful methodology for nursing, we should circumvent the shoals of semantics and accept action research as a metamethodology for nursing (see Holter & Schwartz-Barcott, 1993).

Reluctance to communicate with clients has distinguished the modern medical/pharmaceutical industry in the United States (Fosburg, 1995). Yet it is interesting to note that communication is central to the flourishing arena of alternative therapy: for example, healing as connection or community, or health care via interactive computer program. Action research, enhanced by communicative action, is a collaborative process. Power is shared; there is no place for control or domination. The people—client as individual, group, or community—are ready for action research. Are we?

The economics and politics of a country influence its social systems and professions. Both retrenchment and resurgence characterize the short history of action research. Will methodology for nursing empower nurses to lead, enlist nurses to follow, or enable nurses to get out of the way? Action research, strengthened by communicative action, affirms and advances the scientific, practical, and ethical tenets of contemporary nursing. Action research is authentic methodology for the study of nursing. Action research is a way in which nursing can fulfill its social contract and move confidently into the next century.

REFERENCES

Armitage, P., Chapney-Smith, J., & Andrews, K. (1991). Primary nursing and the role of the nurse preceptor in changing long-term mental health care: An evaluation. *Journal of Advanced Nursing, 16,* 413-422.

Deflem, M. (Ed.). (1996). *Habermas, modernity and law.* London: Sage.

Degerhammar, M., & Wade, B. (1991). The introduction of a new system of care delivery into a surgical ward in Sweden. *International Journal of Nursing Studies, 28,* 325-336.

Ditson, L. A. (1994). Efforts to reduce homemaker/home health aide turnover in a home care agency. *Journal of Home Health Care Practice, 6,* 33-44.

Donaldson, I. (1992). The use of learning contracts in the clinical area. *Nurse Education Today, 12,* 431-436.

Fetterman, D. M. (1995). *Empowerment evaluation.* Thousand Oaks, CA: Sage.

Fosburg, L. (1995, May 19). The world of alternative medicine. *Boston Globe,* p. 21.

Habermas, J. (1984). *The theory of communicative action: Vol.1. Reason and rationalization of society.* Boston: Beacon.

Habermas, J. (1987). *The theory of communicative action: Vol. 2. Lifeworld and system: A critique of functionalist reason.* Boston: Beacon.

Holter, I. M. (1988). Critical theory: A foundation for the development of nursing theories. *Scholarly Inquiry for Nursing Practice, 2,* 223-232.

Holter, I. M., & Schwartz-Barcott, D. (1993). Action research: What is it? How has it been used and how can it be used in nursing? *Journal of Advanced Nursing, 18,* 298-304.

Horkheimer, M. (1972). Traditional and critical theory. In A. Schmidt (Ed.), *Critical theory* (pp. 188-232). New York: Herder & Herder.

Jasper, M. A. (1994). A shortened common foundation programme for graduates: The student's experience of student-centered learning. *Nurse Education Today, 14,* 238-244.

Jillings, C. R. (1992). *Back in circulation, or dancing around the circle? Participatory action research in the context of cardiac rehabilitation.* Unpublished doctoral dissertation, Union Institute, Cincinnati, OH.

Laitinen, P. (1994). Elderly patients' and their informal caregivers' perceptions of care given: The study-control ward design. *Journal of Advanced Nursing, 20,* 71-76.

Lewin, K. (1946). Action research and minority problems. *Journal of Social Issues, 2,* 34-46.

McCaugherty, D. (1991a). The theory-practice gap in nurse education: Its causes and possible solutions. Findings from an action research study. *Journal of Advanced Nursing, 16,* 1055-1061.

McCaugherty, D. (1991b). The use of a teaching model to promote reflection and experiential integration of theory and practice in first-year student nurses: An action research study. *Journal of Advanced Nursing, 16,* 534-543.

Moch, S. D., Roth, D., Pederson, A. Groh-Demers, L., & Siler, J. (1994). Healthier work environments through action research. *Nursing Management, 25,* 38-40.

Newman, M. (1979). *Theory development in nursing.* Philadelphia: F. A. Davis.

Newman, M. (1990). Newman's theory of health as praxis. *Nursing Science Quarterly, 3,* 7-41.

Norman, A. D., & Brandeis, L. (1992). Addressing the needs of survivors: An action approach. *Journal of Psychosocial Oncology, 10,* 3-18.

Ocquist, P. (1978). The epistemology of action research. *Acta Sociologica, 21,* 143-163.

Patton, M. A. (1993). Action research and the process of continual quality improvement in a cancer center. *Oncology Nursing Forum, 20,* 751-755.

Power, F. L., Gillies, P. A., Madeley, R. J., & Abbott, M. (1989). Research in an antenatal clinic: The experience of the Nottingham Mothers' Stop Smoking Project. *Midwifery, 5,* 106-112.

Rasmussen, S. (1984). *Action research for nursing: A unification model.* Unpublished master's thesis, Anna Maria College, Paxton, MA.

Rasmussen, S. (1992, March). *Nursing as communicative process.* Paper presented at the Critical and Feminist Perspectives in Nursing Conference, Toledo, OH.

Rasmussen, S. (1994, May). *Nursing as interactive process.* Paper presented at the International Nursing Research Conference, Vancouver.

Stevens, B. J. (1984). *Nursing theory: Analysis, application, evaluation* (2nd ed.). Boston: Little, Brown.

Susman, G. I., & Evered, R. D. (1978). An assessment of the scientific merits of action research. *Administrative Science Quarterly, 23,* 582-603.

Titchen, A., & Binnie, A. (1993). What am I meant to be doing? Putting practice into theory and back again in new nursing roles. *Journal of Advanced Nursing, 18,* 1054-1065.

Waldow, V. R. (1992). *The conscientization of oppression in Brazilian nursing through feminist pedagogy: A case study.* Unpublished doctoral dissertation, Columbia University Teachers College, New York.

Watts, R. J. (1991). *Rhetoric or reality: A critical analysis of public involvement in the Western Australian health care system.* Unpublished doctoral dissertation, University of Colorado Health Sciences Center, Denver.

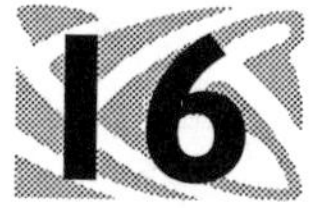

A Feminist Poststructuralist Orientation to Nursing Praxis

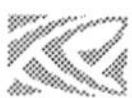

JANICE McCORMICK
JOANNE ROUSSY

Nursing scholars, practitioners, and researchers are increasingly concerned with the social and political implications of nursing science. Not content merely to describe unjust social conditions that adversely affect health, or simply to plan and evaluate interventions designed to assist individuals in adapting to oppressive situations, nurses have turned to a variety of critical, emancipatory, and praxis-oriented perspectives to inform research and practice. These viewpoints include feminist theory, critical theory, poststructuralism, and critical or resistance postmodernisms (Allen, 1987; Dickson, 1990; Kincheloe & McLaren, 1994). Nurses who support these diverse theoretical and political positions have in common a commitment to addressing issues of power in social and cultural practices and a belief in the possibility of an emancipatory praxis.

Despite their commonalities, these perspectives reflect some fundamental contradictions concerning underlying philosophies. The various Marxisms, critical theories, and feminisms are, at their roots, modernist projects steeped in Enlightenment values and assumptions

(Hekman, 1990; Luke & Gore, 1992). The discourses of modernity represent "post-Renaissance Enlightenment-based" modes of thought (Grant, 1993) that proclaim reason as the locus of truth and knowledge, and privilege the scientific method. The predominant discourses of modernity are predicated on the notion of progress—the steady advancement of knowledge in social, cultural, and scientific enterprises leading toward a more enlightened and free society. The foundational grand theories or metanarratives of the Enlightenment depend on overarching theoretical discourses that assume underlying common human traits of "man" that transcend historical and cultural contexts (Best & Kellner, 1991; Hekman, 1990; McLaren, 1995).

Postmodernists have critiqued these positions and the humanist metanarratives that underpin them. The "postmodern turn" in disciplines as diverse as art, film, architecture, literary criticism, and social theory represents a rejection of the foundational truths, metanarratives, and grand theories of the Enlightenment (Lather, 1991; Natoli & Hutcheon, 1993). Poststructural and postmodern theorists contest modernist understandings of rationality, knowledge, and truth as being neutral and objective vehicles of progress and emancipation, and pose the alternative interpretation that such constructs are realized through power and domination (Best & Kellner, 1991).

The loss of faith in foundational truths upon which to ground theoretical claims prompts the central question of this chapter: How can feminist and poststructural theory inform nursing praxis? We argue that feminist and poststructural theoretical positions together offer the necessary grounding for a socially responsible nursing practice, and we explore the implications of a critical nursing praxis for research, theory, and practice.

NURSING PRAXIS AND THE EMANCIPATORY PROJECT

An examination of the literature reveals that the term *praxis* is used in a variety of ways. In its most basic sense, praxis is action, as distinct from theory, but with a mutually informative relationship existing between them. This understanding of the term lacks what we perceive to be a necessary focus on emancipatory social change that provides normative direction for action and reflection. Because we are using *praxis* in a very particular way, we want to discuss our understanding and use of this concept. In its original Aristotelian sense, praxis signified the relationship of universal principles to concrete, particular situations, and involved ethical activities aimed at political action within the larger community (Hoy, 1988). Praxis was appropriated by Marxists as a means of conceptualizing the links between theory for social change and the actions needed to bring about that change (Bernstein, 1971). Feminists incorporated praxis as a central tenet of feminist theory in order to focus attention on the political action needed to bring about changes for women. Thus a commitment to resist domination through direct action can be seen as necessary for emancipatory praxis.

In the 1920s, the theoretical tradition of the Frankfurt school, which came to be known as critical theory, was established. Critical theory attempts to articulate both a comprehensive social theory and a critique of oppressive social structures based on hegemonic power relations. The goal of the various critical theories is emancipation from oppressive conditions that limit autonomy and responsibility (Allen, 1986). This is achieved through the development of theories that incorporate the practical activities needed to bring about change and commitment to political action. Praxis, in this sense, implies a dialectical relationship between theory and practice, with each informing the other in the direction of emancipatory social change (Lather, 1986).

The notion of praxis acknowledges that research and practice are inevitably theory-laden and that these theories are influenced by individuals' ideological commitments. In praxis, nurses become aware of the links among theory, research, and practice. Nursing practice and research become theory-in-action, and practice informs research and theory building. We advocate a *critical* nursing praxis, one that is informed by critical, poststructural, and feminist theoretical perspectives and grounded in ethics, a politics of difference, and a commitment to social justice.

The inclusion of poststructural and postmodern theoretical perspectives in a definition of critical praxis is contested by some critics.

Postmodern and poststructural positions have generated vigorous debate among scholars, social activists, and others concerned with emancipatory praxis. At issue is the fact that humanist notions of social justice, equality, liberty, and individual human rights are bound up with the concept of emancipation, which figures prominently in modernist philosophical, ethical, and political thought (Best & Kellner, 1991; Giroux, 1991; Hekman, 1990; McLaren, 1995). Critics, including many feminists, fear that postmodern and poststructural theories erode the moral grounding of rights-based claims and charge that these positions promote rampant relativism and perpetuate the status quo. These debates create a tension that cannot be ignored by nursing scholars and researchers interested in nursing praxis. Indeed, Reed (1995) has questioned the ability of postmodern theories to form the basis for a critical nursing practice.

Despite these concerns, we argue that a feminist poststructural perspective offers powerful theoretical tools to enable nurses to uncover the power imbalances and vested interests in the everyday, taken-for-granted operations of society. We will show that charges of relativism are unfounded and that feminist poststructuralism can inform a critical nursing praxis. In the next sections, we examine these theoretical underpinnings and address the criticisms that have been raised.

POSTSTRUCTURALISM

Best and Kellner (1991) characterize poststructuralism as a type of postmodern theory, arguing that poststructuralism is a "subset of a broader range of theoretical, cultural and social tendencies which constitute postmodern discourses" (p. 25). The poststructuralist critique centers on a rejection of structuralist thinking that reasserts modernist notions of truth, objectivity, and certainty. Far from being a unified theory, poststructuralism includes diverse theoretical positions, including those found in important works by Derrida, Baudrillard, Lyotard, Kristeva, and Foucault (Best & Kellner, 1991). We rely on Foucault's theories of discourse, subjectivity, knowledge, and power in our explication of poststructuralism.

The core of Foucault's theories includes (a) the rejection of modernist notions of grand narratives, especially the humanist metanarrative; (b) the rejection of the essentialism of modernism; (c) an emphasis on the notion of difference and multivocality; (d) a preoccupation with language and discourse, especially with discursive practices that are implicated in the construction of subjectivities; (e) a claim that knowledge and power are inevitably linked through discourse and that the dominant discourses of a society produce and reproduce "truth" that benefits powerful social groups; and (f) an assertion that the disciplines represent dominant discourses that produce subjectivities, knowledge, and, therefore, power (Best & Kellner, 1991; Diamond & Quinby, 1988; Hekman, 1990; Weedon, 1987).

One of Foucault's most notable contributions to social criticism is his insight that knowledge and power are inextricably linked in discourse. A poststructural conception of power is one in which discourse is the medium through which power relations are maintained and reproduced, and through which identities are constituted. Foucault (1976/1990) declares that power is everywhere, comes from everywhere, cannot be "possessed, held, acquired, seized or shared, but only exercised" (p. 92).

Foucault's critiques reveal fresh insights for feminists and other scholars by demonstrating how power and discourse have operated in society in specific historical periods and contexts. However, although he exposes how discourses and practices have served as "regimes of truth," Foucault refuses to comment in his work on preferred uses of power or to discuss methods for changing prevailing discourses. Thus a criticism of the poststructuralist perspective is that the perceived lack of direction for change will result in a social science content to deconstruct texts without changing the status quo (McLaren, 1995). For this reason, postmodern and poststructural perspectives have sparked passionate responses from several groups, including feminists, the disabled, people of color, antipoverty groups, and gays and lesbians. The concern expressed by such groups is that postmodern critiques will dissolve the liberal humanist philosophy underpinning the discourses of individual rights.

Various theorists, scholars, and political activists have responded to these criticisms with proposed alternative readings of postmodern theories. Politically committed postmodernists and poststructuralists advocate a critical appropriation of postmodern theory as a basis for a socially transformative praxis. Lather (1991), for example, claims, "The various feminisms, neo-Marxisms and some of the poststructuralisms . . . become kinds of critical theories which are informed by identification with and interest in oppositional social movements" (p. 3). Giroux (1991) proposes that the discourses of postmodernism, feminism, and those emancipatory discourses of modernism that champion human freedom and social justice represent three of the most important theoretical stances for creating a renewed cultural politics.

In another reply to critics, postmodern scholars have distinguished among different strands of postmodernism. Thus Ebert (1991) identifies two basic types of postmodernism: ludic and resistance postmodernisms. In *ludic postmodernism,* as theorized by Lyotard, Derrida, and Baudrillard, politics becomes a "textual practice [of] parody, pastiche, and fragmentation that unsettles, decenters, and disrupts rather than transforms the totalizing circulation of meaning within grand narratives and dominant discursive apparatuses" (McLaren, 1995, p. 207). The effect is an "endless play of signification" resulting in the essential undecidability of meaning. *Resistance* or *critical postmodernisms* are appropriations and extensions of ludic postmodernism that include a "materialist intervention" based on incorporating social and historical factors into a "meaningful critique of social practices and power" (p. 208). The resulting theoretical perspectives are capable of exposing the inconsistencies and incongruities in the rules by which we order our existing social arrangements.

The positions taken by some who argue against poststructuralism and postmodernism are extreme in that they do not acknowledge the reservations and exceptions many theorists have incorporated into their writings. As Code (1991) has argued, the important issues that postmodernism raises (issues of power, knowledge, truth, and how dominant discourses are implicated in the creation of desire and subjectivity) tend to get lost in a general attack on relativism, irrationality, and nihilism. Historically, the debate between relativism and objectivity has been constructed as a struggle between binary opposites. This false dichotomy forces individuals into rigid polarities that fail to uncover the complexities inherent in each position. Divisions such as culture/nature, rational/irrational, mind/body, and male/female reflect hierarchical differences in power, with one term clearly superior to the other. It should be noted, however, that the "superior" term derives its status and meaning *through* being contrasted with its opposite in such binary couplings.

Rather than engaging in these "either/or" positions, Code (1991) proposes a middle ground that recognizes knowledge as perspectival and located in historical contexts. This position incorporates what is best in theoretical and practical positions and rejects "what is damaging and oppressive" (p. 318). Adopting this approach expands the options available to practitioners, who can incorporate aspects of various theoretical perspectives to compensate for gaps and omissions in each. Such theoretical partnerships include feminist poststructuralism. Feminists have engaged in sustained debates on the merits and dangers that postmodern and poststructuralist theories represent for emancipatory practice and have thoughtfully considered how feminist theory can productively incorporate aspects of these positions while retaining their orientation toward praxis. It is to these debates that we now turn.

FEMINIST POSTSTRUCTURALISM

Interest in feminist and poststructuralist theoretical perspectives has been growing in the nursing literature (Cheek & Rudge, 1994a, 1994b; Dickson, 1990; Dzurec, 1989; May, 1992). Several feminist scholars have noted the compatibility of poststructuralist theories with much of feminist thought. For example, both challenge the anthropocentric definition of knowledge, both reject notions of a universal voice and instead opt for polyvocality, both are concerned with the idea of difference and with the "other" and how these ideas are theorized, both identify the body as the site of power, and both focus on discourse and issues of power, hierarchy, and hegemony (Bell, 1993; Diamond & Quinby, 1988; Hekman, 1990). Notwithstanding these similarities, there is not necessarily a "happy marriage" between poststructuralism and feminism (Diamond & Quinby, 1988). For example, feminists have noted a lack of attention to gender or feminist issues in the work of many poststructuralists. Moreover, the perceived lack of normative direction in postmodern and poststructuralist theory is contrary to feminist aims to bring about change in existing power arrangements. For these reasons, many feminists have argued for the inclusion of feminist perspectives in poststructuralist theories and in research using these theories (Luke & Gore, 1992). These feminists have cautiously appropriated aspects of poststructural theories of power, language, and subjectivity that offer strategic advantages for the construction of emancipatory feminist theory.

Weedon (1987) defines feminist poststructuralism as "a mode of knowledge production which uses poststructuralist theories of language, subjectivity, social processes and institutions to understand existing power relations and to identify areas and strategies for change" (pp. 40-41). Important tenets of this perspective include the view that knowledge is socially produced and that subjectivities are constituted discursively through language and discourse. A central concern is with the issue of power and how language and social practices serve to perpetuate imbalances of power in society.

It should be noted that Weedon's definition stresses the theoretical principles of poststructuralism and does not address feminist theoretical perspectives. Other theorists have attended to the ways in which a specifically feminist application of poststructural theories differs from forms of poststructural theorizing that are not feminist (Diamond & Quinby, 1988; Luke & Gore, 1992). While valuing the utility of the poststructuralist theoretical tools, many feminist poststructuralists are cautious about accepting the antifoundationalism of poststructuralism, arguing that a foundation based on feminist principles provides the necessary grounding for feminists committed to changing the status quo. Luke and Gore (1992) claim that because this foundation rests on a politics of difference in subject location, identity, and knowledge, it is antiessentialist. The feminist commitment to political action, social change, and praxis gives feminist poststructuralism the action orientation that nurses need to create a critical nursing practice—one that is committed to challenging existing institutional and disciplinary arrangements that disempower, limit freedom and agency, and unfairly distribute human and social goods, such as health.

How can feminist poststructuralist principles inform nursing praxis? One way is through the incorporation of these principles into nursing research and theorizing. In the following sections we explore some of the ways this can be done and speculate on the benefits for nursing praxis.

IMPLICATIONS OF A FEMINIST POSTSTRUCTURALIST PERSPECTIVE: NURSING RESEARCH

At the heart of feminist research is the notion of praxis. Lather (1986) refers to "research as praxis," in which researchers attempt not only to understand and critique the power imbalances in society, but also to "change that maldistribution to help create a more equal world" (p. 258). Research as praxis is a method for creating knowledge relevant for social policy and helping to change the lives of those who are locked into unfair or oppressive social structures. Nursing research informed by a feminist poststructuralist perspective is research with a political agenda. Researchers and scholars who hold such views are committed to developing knowledge that can contribute to social, political, and economic changes in the structures of society that affect health and illness. Such knowledge and critique are grounded in an awareness of the sociopolitical realities and historical contexts of the lives of individuals. This awareness sensitizes researchers to the pervasive effects of power relationships and taken-for-granted practices that perpetuate these relations. A feminist poststructuralist perspective provides a critical framework from which to view and analyze the world.

Both feminism and poststructuralism have implications for how nurses approach research. Feminist critiques of science and the nature of reality, truth, verification, and knowledge are core issues in feminist scholarship. Together with a prevailing concern with power relationships, these central concepts have had a profound impact on how feminists conceptualize the research enterprise. Many of these critiques of science have focused on a sustained attack on the philosophical underpinnings of the dominant view of science referred to as logical positivism (Bleier, 1989). Feminists and other scholars have convincingly argued against the possibility of value-free theory and theory-free observation (Harding, 1991). In considering the project of social research, poststructuralists also challenge the notion of objectivity; the value-free or value-neutral stance of the researcher toward the questions, methods, subjects, and interpretations of research; and the relationship between the researcher and the researched. Feminist researchers require strong reflexivity; they must reflect on how their own values, beliefs, and experiences influence their choices of research methods, questions, and methodology, as well as on how interactions between researchers and participants affect the data that are collected and how they are interpreted.

Nurse researchers who subscribe to a feminist poststructuralist perspective approach inquiry with specific understandings about the relationships they expect to have with the participants in their studies. Feminist researchers have criticized hierarchical relationships between the researcher and the researched wherein the researched are deceived, manipulated, or simply used for the data they can provide, with no provision for reciprocity. Feminist poststructuralist researchers are sensitive to the potential for abuse of power in the researcher-participant relationship, and they attempt to build in safeguards against such abuse. For example, feminist researchers have approached the qualitative research interview in unique ways. Rather than seeing the interview as simply a means of obtaining information as quickly and efficiently as possible, feminist researchers reflexively study the nature of the relationship between themselves and research participants and how this affects the knowledge that is constructed (Anderson, 1991; Oakley, 1981).

The research interview can be seen as a kind of "confessional." Foucault (1976/1990) characterizes confession as one of the primary techniques used in the production of truth: "The confession is a ritual of discourse in which the speaking subject is also the subject of the statement; it is also a ritual that unfolds within a power relationship" (p. 61). The research interview can be seen as an example of a confession in that the researcher holds the power of interpreting the meaning of the words and stories spoken by the participant; in other words, she or he creates "truth" from them. For this reason, it is essential that the feminist poststructuralist researcher build in procedures to prevent this unwarranted use of power over participants. The use of member checks (Lincoln & Guba, 1985) is one way of accomplishing this. Member checks can take different forms, from simply providing participants with the transcripts of interviews to allowing participants to change or interpret their utterances (Mishler, 1986).

Above all, a feminist poststructural perspective can influence research by fostering a sensitivity to differences: first, an awareness of how our own subject positions affect our research interests, the selection of research participants, and the resultant knowledge that is constructed; second, a realization of the intersecting nature of sexism, racism, classism, and other forms of oppression makes visible the unwritten rules of exclusion that operate in society. For example, feminists have argued for the inclusion of gender as a category of analysis. The ideological goals of feminist research are to make women visible and to end the distortion of female experiences as a means of ending women's unequal status in patriarchal society. Making gender a category of analysis in research is a fundamental approach to uncovering the ways that gender is implicated in the taken-for-granted operations of social institutions. Silva (1994) refers to a gender lens, that is, a lens through which we can more clearly understand what is missing in our priorities, theories, categories of analysis, and strategies. This feminist re-visioning can transform disciplines by calling into question the basic concepts, orienting assumptions, theoretical frameworks, and paradigms upon which members of the discipline build knowledge (Stacey & Thorne, 1985).

What implications does feminist poststructuralism have for nursing theory? What might such nursing theory look like, and what difference would it make for nurses, nursing, and the health of individuals?

NURSING THEORY

A feminist poststructuralist perspective leads us to challenge the foundational "truths" that are central to a discipline. We are encouraged to problematize what we consider to be knowledge and how this knowledge is constructed, to interrogate the processes by which we identify the phenomena central to our discipline, and to reflect on which questions get asked and which ignored. Both feminist and poststructuralist theories demand a rethinking of our basic assumptions about gender, power, truth, knowledge, and the very nature of institutions and disciplines (Weedon, 1987).

So-called grand theories or metanarratives are conceptual models or maps that are developed to account for the organization of social behavior over time. However, a universally applicable theory cannot account for the historical and cultural context in which all observation is embedded, and therefore does not exist in the real world. The grand narratives in nursing can be considered to be the 20 or so major nursing theories that were created almost exclusively in North America from the 1950s to the 1980s. Nursing theories are products of the historical, social, and political contexts in which they originated. What is unacknowledged is that these theories are creations of actual embodied individuals within specific times and locations. As such, they reflect cultural assumptions that privilege educated, white, middle-class, and Western (overwhelmingly American) perspectives.

A feminist poststructural perspective in nursing theory would encourage the examination of the assumptions underlying theoretical constructs and consider how nursing theories function to create, reproduce, or challenge power imbalances. Such a reexamination might, for example, retain the metaparadigm concepts of health, environment, person, and nursing as useful heuristic devices within a feminist poststructuralist re-visioning of nursing theory. However, they would, in all likelihood, encompass the broader context of the social, economic, and contextual variables that affect health rather than focus on individual and psychological variables alone. Furthermore, feminist poststructuralist nursing theories would direct the nurse to consider how gender, class, race, sexual orientation, and other subject locations are implicated in the ways individuals experience health, illness, and health care services. The danger of rejecting the invitation that postmodernism and poststructuralism provide to reconceptualize theoretical positions is that we will fail to address the role of power in nursing and continue to ignore issues of racism, classism, sexism, heterosexism, and ageism in nursing education, practice, research, and theorizing.

Nursing cannot function without normative direction; it does not follow, however, that such direction must necessarily be provided by grand theories or metanarratives. To reject the possibility of a transcendent truth is not to imply relativism or the impossibility of normative directions. It is our view that we must be wary of a premature acceptance of metatheoretical conceptualizations. Such positionings avoid the necessary interrogation of these conceptualizations and risk reifying them. Theories are necessary tools that enable us to construct knowledge for selected purposes. They describe and reflect aspects of the world, but they underdetermine the variability and complexity that exist. Nurses who have a commitment to critical nursing praxis recognize the importance of theoretical perspectives that help expose the power and hierarchy embedded in the social world in which health care decisions are made.

We have described critical nursing praxis as a triad consisting of a theoretical perspective based on feminist, poststructural, and critical theories; nursing research activities informed by these theoretical perspectives; and, finally, practice that incorporates emancipatory values, critical theoretical perspectives, and knowledge from nursing research. In the final section we discuss how these components influence nursing praxis and offer some examples of praxis.

TOWARD A FEMINIST POSTSTRUCTURALIST NURSING PRAXIS

Feminist poststructuralism offers a way of theorizing the nature of power, how it functions in health care disciplines and institutions, and how nurses are both subjected to and implicated in disciplinary uses of power. This perspective encourages nurses to reconceptualize the project of nursing research, to problematize the methodologies and ethics of research and the politics of which questions get asked and which do not. A feminist poststructural perspective also provides the basis for a critique of nursing theory and nursing power. A critique informed by feminist (DeMarco, Campbell, & Wuest, 1993) and poststructuralist perspectives provides a lens to enable nurses to "see" androcentric, ethnocentric, and class bias in our theories, knowledge base, and research approaches. However, because nursing is a practice profession, it is not enough for nurses simply to critique and deconstruct social theories. Criticism that is not connected to comprehensive recommendations and plans for action is incapable of changing the status quo.

Nurses who conceive of their practice as critical nursing praxis challenge the naturalness of the social order they encounter. They use theoretical perspectives on power and domination to redefine health care issues as the outcomes of specific policy decisions, rather than as inevitable consequences of individual choice. These understandings make nurses unwilling simply to encourage clients to "cope" with social and economic conditions that disempower and oppress them. Moreover, nurses learn to question explanations that locate responsibility for illness and health at the level of the individual alone. The notion of a critical nursing praxis means that nurses examine how decisions made at the larger social, political, and economic levels of society affect their clients and themselves at the local level. For example, although nurses work with the health needs of specific individuals, they incorporate a concern for the determinants of health and illness beyond the level of the individual. Nurse activists have demonstrated that environmental, political, and economic decisions occurring at the macro level of society have profound impacts on the health of individuals (Butterfield, 1990; Chopoorian, 1986; Stevens, 1989). These decisions also have impacts on the provision of nursing care within the health care system in which most nurses work. Using these perspectives to uncover and critique unjust social practices enables nurses to change the way they interact with individual clients and to work toward changes at the policy level. By such actions, nurses can interrupt the hegemonic discourses within nursing that maintain existing social arrangements.

The theoretical perspectives that underpin nursing research directly influence the nursing knowledge that results and thus have impacts on patient care. We must examine carefully what the potential effects of such theoretical positions will be for clients and communities. At the same time, we need to be cognizant of how such stances position nursing socially and politically to effect changes that will benefit the health of populations. The knowledge we generate has social and political consequences for the people we serve and for the discipline of nursing. A commitment to praxis demands that we continually monitor and evaluate these social effects to determine how well they coincide with our vision, values, and goals. Attempting to avoid consideration of the social and political implications of nursing actions is not a neutral stance; such a decision endorses the status quo and supports existing power arrangements. As individuals and as professionals committed to health and healing, we need to ask, What are the health implications of the knowledge we create, and who benefits?

Although the search for solid positions on which to ground knowledge and theory construction seems a reasonable quest in a shifting and turbulent world, we have slowly and uncomfortably come to realize that this is a false and untenable objective. There is no Archimedean point, no fixed location in the universe upon which we can ground our theories. Instead of discovering universal truths, we create knowledge that is tentative, contextual, and physically and historically situated. Critical theories informed by feminist and poststructuralist perspectives can help us challenge the inequalities that threaten the health of individuals and communities. Further, they enable us to address our theorizing and practice to larger social and political processes—to engage, in other words, in critical nursing praxis.

REFERENCES

Allen, D. G. (1986). Using philosophical and historical methodologies to understand the concept of health. In P. L. Chinn (Ed.), *Nursing research methodology: Issues and implementation* (pp. 157-168). Rockville, MD: Aspen.

Allen, D. G. (1987). Critical social theory as a model for analyzing ethical issues in family and community health. *Family and Community Health, 10*(1), 63-72.

Anderson, J. M. (1991). Reflexivity in fieldwork: Toward a feminist epistemology. *Image: The Journal of Nursing Scholarship, 23,* 115-118.

Bell, D. (1993). Introduction 1: The context. In D. Bell, P. Caplan, & W. J. Karim (Eds.), *Gendered fields: Women, men and ethnography* (pp. 1-18). London: Routledge.

Bernstein, R. J. (1971). *Praxis and action: Contemporary philosophies of human activity.* Philadelphia: University of Pennsylvania Press.

Best, S., & Kellner, D. (1991). *Postmodern theory: Critical interrogations.* New York: Guilford.

Bleier, R. (Ed.). (1989). *Feminist approaches to science.* New York: Teachers College Press.

Butterfield, P. G. (1990). Thinking upstream: Nurturing a conceptual understanding of the societal context of health behavior. *Advances in Nursing Science, 12*(2), 1-8.

Cheek, J., & Rudge, T. (1994a). The panopticon revisited? An exploration of the social and political dimensions of contemporary health care and nursing practice. *International Journal of Nursing Studies, 31*, 583-591.

Cheek, J., & Rudge, T. (1994b). Webs of documentation: The discourse of case notes. *Australian Journal of Communication, 21*(2), 41-52.

Chopoorian, T. J. (1986). Reconceptualizing the environment. In P. Moccia (Ed.), *New approaches to theory development* (pp. 39-54). New York: National League for Nursing.

Code, L. (1991). *What can she know? Feminist theory and the construction of knowledge.* Ithaca, NY: Cornell University Press.

DeMarco, R., Campbell, J., & Wuest, J. (1993). Feminist critique: Searching for meaning in research. *Advances in Nursing Science, 16*(2), 26-38.

Diamond, I., & Quinby, L. (Eds.). (1988). *Feminism and Foucault: Reflections of resistance.* Boston: Northeastern University Press.

Dickson, G. L. (1990). A feminist poststructuralist analysis of the knowledge of menopause. *Advances in Nursing Science, 12*(3), 15-31.

Dzurec, L. C. (1989). The necessity for and evolution of multiple paradigms for nursing research: A poststructuralist perspective. *Advances in Nursing Science, 11*(4), 69-77.

Ebert, T. (1991). Writing in the political: Resistance (post)modernism. *Legal Studies Forum, 15*, 291-303.

Foucault, M. (1990). *The history of sexuality: Vol. 1. An introduction* (R. Hurley, Trans.). New York: Vintage. (Original work published 1976)

Giroux, H. A. (Ed.). (1991). *Postmodernism, feminism, and cultural politics: Redrawing educational boundaries.* Albany: State University of New York Press.

Grant, J. (1993). *Fundamental feminism: Contesting the core concepts of feminist theory.* New York: Routledge.

Harding, S. (1991). *Whose science? Whose knowledge? Thinking from women's lives.* New York: Cornell University Press.

Hekman, S. J. (1990). *Gender and knowledge: Elements of a postmodern feminism.* Boston: Northeastern University Press.

Hoy, T. (1988). *Praxis, truth and liberation: Essays on Gadamer, Taylor, Polanyi, Habermas, Gutierrez, and Ricoeur.* Lanham, MD: University Press of America.

Kincheloe, J. L., & McLaren, P. L. (1994). Rethinking critical theory and qualitative research. In N. K. Denzin & Y. S. Lincoln (Eds.), *Handbook of qualitative research* (pp. 138-157). Thousand Oaks, CA: Sage.

Lather, P. (1986). Research as praxis. *Harvard Educational Review, 56*, 257-276.

Lather, P. (1991). *Getting smart: Feminist research and pedagogy with/in the postmodern.* New York: Routledge.

Lincoln, Y. S., & Guba, E. G. (1985). *Naturalistic inquiry.* Beverly Hills, CA: Sage.

Luke, C., & Gore, J. (Eds.). (1992). *Feminisms and critical pedagogy.* New York: Routledge.

May, C. (1992). Individual care? Power and subjectivity in therapeutic relationships. *Sociology, 26*, 589-602.

McLaren, P. (1995). *Critical pedagogy and predatory culture.* London: Routledge.

Mishler, E. G. (1986). *Research interviewing: Context and narrative.* Cambridge, MA: Harvard University Press.

Natoli, J. P., & Hutcheon, L. (Eds.). (1993). *A postmodern reader.* Albany: State University of New York Press.

Oakley, A. (1981). Interviewing women: A contradiction in terms. In H. Roberts (Ed.), *Doing feminist research* (pp. 30-61). London: Routledge & Kegan Paul.

Reed, P. G. (1995). A treatise on nursing knowledge development for the 21st century: Beyond postmodernism. *Advances in Nursing Science, 17*(3), 70-84.

Silva, N. (1994). Toward a feminist methodology in research on battered women. In A. J. Dan (Ed.), *Reframing women's health: Multidisciplinary research and practice* (pp. 290-298). Thousand Oaks, CA: Sage.

Stacey, J., & Thorne, B. (1985). The missing feminist revolution in sociology. *Social Problems, 32,* 301-316.

Stevens, P. E. (1989). A critical social reconceptualization of environment in nursing: Implications for methodology. *Advances in Nursing Science, 11*(4), 56-68.

Weedon, C. (1987). *Feminist practice and poststructuralist theory.* Oxford, UK: Basil Blackwell.

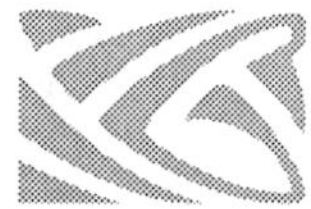

Name Index

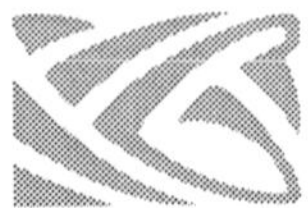

Subject Index

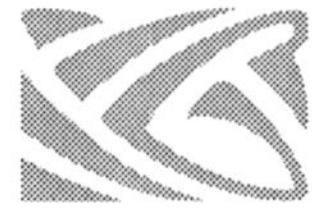

About the Authors

Emília L. Saporiti Angerami, RN, PhD, is Full Research Professor and former Dean of the College of Nursing at Ribeirão Preto University of São Paulo, Brazil, which is a World Health Organization collaborating center for the development of nursing research. She is an expert member of the WHO Panel on Nursing, an international consultant and speaker, and the author of several papers in three languages.

Francisco A. Correia, DPh, is Professor in the Department of Psychiatric Nursing and Human Sciences at the College of Nursing at Ribeirão Preto University of São Paulo, Brazil, which is a World Health Organization collaborating center for the development of nursing research. He is also a lecturer in nursing history, ethics, and bioethics there.

F. Ndidi U. Griffin, RN, CFNP, EdD, is Associate Professor and Graduate Program Director in the Department of Nursing, School of Health and Social Work, California State University, Fresno. She has previously published in the areas of cultural diversity and health care delivery, and her research interests lie in the areas of access to health care and the advancement of a multicultural workforce to meet the needs of a diverse patient population.

Sigrídur Halldórsdóttir, RN, DrMedSci, is Dean of the Faculty of Health Sciences at the University of Akureyri in Iceland. She obtained her master's degree in nursing at the University of British Columbia, and she has recently defended her doctorate in the Department of Caring Sciences at the University of Linköping, Sweden. She is an active educator, researcher, and leader in the area of caring, and has had numerous publications in the field.

Virginia E. Hayes, RN, PhD, is Assistant Professor in the School of Nursing at the University of British Columbia. Her research program centers on the impact of chronic conditions within families, and she teaches courses in family nursing, the nursing of children, and research. She has had a number of publications in the areas of families and pediatric chronicity and family research methods.

Dorothy J. Henderson, RN, PhD, is Assistant Professor in Psychosocial and Community Health in the School of Nursing, University of Washington, Seattle. She is also an adjunct faculty member with the Women's Studies Department at the University of Washington. Her practice, research, and teaching include a strong emphasis on women's mental health, and are grounded in feminist and critical theories. Her research, which uses participatory methodologies, focuses on women's substance abuse.

Joy L. Johnson, RN, PhD, is Assistant Professor in the School of Nursing and Doctoral Research Fellow at the Institute of Health Promotion, University of British Columbia. Her work has focused on philosophical issues related to nursing. Additionally, she has developed a program of research in the field of health promotion, with a particular emphasis on its actualization within clinical settings. She has published numerous chapters and articles in both of these areas.

Marion Jones, RGON, MEd, is a doctoral candidate at Massey University, Palmerson, New Zealand. She is also Principal Lecturer, School of Nursing and Midwifery, and Programme Leader, Master of Health Science, Faculty of Health Studies, Auckland Institute of Technology. She is highly involved in the New Zealand Nurses Association and the National Education Committee for Theatre Nurses and acts as a monitor for degree programs for the New Zealand Qualifications Authority.

Joan Liaschenko, RN, PhD, is a postdoctoral fellow in the School of Nursing, University of California, San Francisco. Her research and publications focus on ethics and the philosophy of nursing practice. She has recently accepted a position as Assistant Professor in the School of Nursing, Department of Health Maintenance, University of Wisconsin—Milwaukee.

Lynne E. Maxwell, RN, MSN, is a doctoral candidate in the School of Nursing, University of British Columbia, and a Lecturer at the School of Nursing, University of Victoria, British Columbia. Her research interests center on health promotion and families, and she is actively involved in several professional organizations promoting cardiovascular health at the local and national levels.

Janice McCormick, RN, MSN, is a doctoral candidate at the University of British Columbia School of Nursing. Her dissertation research is an ethnography investigating how nurses, chronically ill adolescents, and their family members negotiate control over care. She has an extensive clinical background in nephrology nursing and an interest in feminist and poststructural perspectives on power.

Suellen Miller, RN, PhD, is Pew Postdoctoral Research Fellow at the Institute for Health Policy Studies, School of Medicine, University of California, San Francisco. She is actively interested in women's health as a clinical nurse-midwife, educator, international maternal child health consultant, and researcher, bringing a feminist postmodern perspective to her teaching, consulting, practice, research activities, and publications.

Sandra Rasmussen, RN, LMHC, CAS, PhD, is Associate Professor, Department of Nursing, Rhode Island College; Senior Clinician/ Supervisor, New Bedford Child and Family Service; and Senior Instructor, Graduate Program in Counseling Psychology, Cambridge College. She has taught in vocational, undergraduate, and graduate nursing programs in the United States, and has practiced, developed programs, and conducted research in mental health and addiction services.

Pamela A. Ratner, RN, PhD, is Medical Research Council of Canada and Izaak Walton Killam Postdoctoral Research Fellow at the Institute of Health Promotion Research, University of British Columbia. She has directed much of her research activity toward the problems of interpersonal violence and women's health issues from a public health perspective. She is known for her expertise in theory testing and maintains an interest in nursing knowledge development.

Patricia Rodney, RN, MSN, is currently a doctoral candidate at the University of British Columbia School of Nursing, a member of the Executive of the Canadian Bioethics Society, and a Research Associate with the University of British Columbia Centre for Applied Ethics. In addition, she is a Visiting Lecturer at the University of Victoria School of Nursing. Her dissertation research is a feminist, ethnographic study of nurses' enactment of their moral agency within an institutional context. She speaks and publishes widely on nursing ethics.

Joanne Roussy, RN, MSc, is a doctoral candidate in nursing at the University of British Columbia. Her research focuses on the implications of poverty for the health of pregnant women.

Margarete Sandelowski, RN, PhD, FAAN, is Professor in the Department of Women's and Children's Health in the School of Nursing at the University of North Carolina at Chapel Hill. She has published extensively in nursing and social science journals and anthologies on the subjects of reproductive technology, technology in nursing, infertility, and qualitative methods, and is the author of three books, including the award-winning *With Child in Mind: Studies of the Personal Encounter with Infertility* (1993). She is currently working on a social history of technology in nursing.

Rosalie Starzomski, RN, MN, is Nephrology/Transplant Clinical Nurse Specialist, Visiting Lecturer in the School of Nursing at the University of Victoria, British Columbia, and a doctoral candidate in the School of Nursing at the University of British Columbia. Her research and publications are focused on ethics, health policy, nephrology nursing, and organ transplantation. She holds a joint appointment at the Vancouver Hospital and Health Sciences Center as an ethics consultant and teaches ethics across disciplines.

Sally E. Thorne, RN, PhD, is Associate Professor in the School of Nursing at the University of British Columbia. Her research into the intersection between chronic illness experience and health service delivery has been published in various arenas, including a recent book. Currently she teaches graduate courses in the philosophy of nursing science and maintains an active involvement in injecting nursing's voice into health policy.

Donna M. Trainor, RN, EdD, is Director of Nursing and Associate Professor of Nursing and Psychology, Massachusetts College of Pharmacy and Allied Health Sciences. She is active on a number of state, regional, and national academic boards and committees and consults regularly in the area of nursing management and education. Her research centers on the philosophy of nursing, theoretical analysis, and cognition and epistemology as they pertain to nursing education.

Colleen Varcoe, RN, MEd, MSN, is a doctoral candidate in nursing at the University of British Columbia School of Nursing. She also teaches at the British Columbia Institute of Technology in the Nursing Specialties, especially in critical care, emergency, and nephrology nursing. She has published in the areas of knowledge-based nursing practice, research utilization, and power relations, and is investigating these areas in relation to nursing's contribution to ending violence against women.